HEALTH LITERACY
AND CONSUMER-FACING TECHNOLOGY

WORKSHOP SUMMARY

Joe Alper, *Rapporteur*

Roundtable on Health Literacy

Board on Population Health and Public Health Practice

Institute of Medicine

The National Academies of
SCIENCES · ENGINEERING · MEDICINE

THE NATIONAL ACADEMIES PRESS
Washington, DC
www.nap.edu

THE NATIONAL ACADEMIES PRESS   500 Fifth Street, NW   Washington, DC 20001

This activity was supported by contracts between the National Academy of Sciences and the Aetna Foundation; the Agency for Healthcare Research and Quality (HHSP233200900537P); Bristol-Myers Squibb; California Dental Association; East Bay Community Foundation (Kaiser Permanente); Eli Lilly and Company; Health Literacy Missouri; Health Literacy Partners; Health Resources and Services Administration (HHSH25034004T); Humana; Institute for Healthcare Advancement; Merck & Co., Inc.; National Institutes of Health; North Shore–Long Island Jewish Health System; Office of Disease Prevention and Health Promotion; and UnitedHealth Group. The views presented in this publication do not necessarily reflect the views of the organizations or agencies that provided support for the activity.

International Standard Book Number-13: 978-0-309-37690-7
International Standard Book Number-10: 0-309-37690-4

Additional copies of this workshop summary are available for sale from the National Academies Press, 500 Fifth Street, NW, Keck 360, Washington, DC 20001; (800) 624-6242 or (202) 334-3313; http://www.nap.edu.

Copyright 2015 by the National Academy of Sciences. All rights reserved.

Printed in the United States of America

Suggested citation: National Academies of Sciences, Engineering, and Medicine. 2015. *Health literacy and consumer-facing technology: Workshop summary.* Washington, DC: The National Academies Press.

The National Academies of
SCIENCES · ENGINEERING · MEDICINE

The **National Academy of Sciences** was established in 1863 by an Act of Congress, signed by President Lincoln, as a private, nongovernmental institution to advise the nation on issues related to science and technology. Members are elected by their peers for outstanding contributions to research. Dr. Ralph J. Cicerone is president.

The **National Academy of Engineering** was established in 1964 under the charter of the National Academy of Sciences to bring the practices of engineering to advising the nation. Members are elected by their peers for extraordinary contributions to engineering. Dr. C. D. Mote, Jr., is president.

The **National Academy of Medicine** (formerly the Institute of Medicine) was established in 1970 under the charter of the National Academy of Sciences to advise the nation on medical and health issues. Members are elected by their peers for distinguished contributions to medicine and health. Dr. Victor J. Dzau is president.

The three Academies work together as the **National Academies of Sciences, Engineering, and Medicine** to provide independent, objective analysis and advice to the nation and conduct other activities to solve complex problems and inform public policy decisions. The Academies also encourage education and research, recognize outstanding contributions to knowledge, and increase public understanding in matters of science, engineering, and medicine.

Learn more about the National Academies of Sciences, Engineering, and Medicine at **www.national-academies.org**.

PLANNING COMMITTEE ON HEALTH LITERACY AND CONSUMER-FACING TECHNOLOGY[1]

SUZANNE BAKKEN, Alumni Professor of Nursing and Professor of Biomedical Informatics, Columbia University School of Nursing
GILLIAN CHRISTIE, Health Innovation Analyst, The Vitality Institute
GARTH GRAHAM, President, Aetna Foundation
LINDA HARRIS, Division Director, Health Communication and eHealth Team, U.S. Department of Health and Human Services
PAMELA JEFFRIES, Vice Provost for Digital Initiatives, Johns Hopkins University
ANDREW PLEASANT, Senior Director for Health Literacy and Research, Canyon Ranch Institute
TED VICKEY, Founder and President, FitWell, Inc.

---

[1] Institute of Medicine planning committees are solely responsible for organizing the workshop, identifying topics, and choosing speakers. The responsibility for the published workshop summary rests with the workshop rapporteur and the institution.

ROUNDTABLE ON HEALTH LITERACY[1]

BERNARD ROSOF (*Chair*), Chief Executive Officer, Quality in Healthcare Advisory Group, LLC
MARIN P. ALLEN, Deputy Associate Director for Communications and Public Liaison and Director of Public Information, National Institutes of Health
WILMA ALVARADO-LITTLE, Principal and Founder, Alvarado-Little Consulting, LLC
SUZANNE BAKKEN, Alumni Professor of Nursing and Professor of Biomedical Informatics, Columbia University
CINDY BRACH, Senior Health Policy Researcher, Agency for Healthcare Research and Quality
GEM DAUS, Public Health Analyst, Health Resources and Services Administration
TERRY DAVIS, Professor of Medicine and Pediatrics, Louisiana State University Health Sciences Center
CHRISTOPHER DEZII, Director, Healthcare Quality and Performance Measures, Bristol-Myers Squibb Company
JENNIFER DILLAHA, Medical Director for Immunizations, Medical Advisor, Health Literacy and Communication, Arkansas Department of Health
ALICIA FERNANDEZ, Professor of Clinical Medicine, University of California, San Francisco
LAURIE FRANCIS, Senior Director of Clinic Operations and Quality, Oregon Primary Care Association
GARTH GRAHAM, President, Aetna Founation
LORI HALL, Consultant, Health Education, Eli Lilly and Company
LINDA HARRIS, Division Director, Health Communication and eHealth Team, U.S. Department of Health and Human Services
BETSY L. HUMPHREYS, Deputy Director, National Library of Medicine
MARGARET LOVELAND, Senior Director, Global Medical Affairs, Merck & Co.
LAURIE MYERS, Leader of Health Literacy Strategy, Merck & Co.
CATINA O'LEARY, President and Chief Executive Officer, Health Literacy Missouri
MICHAEL PAASCHE-ORLOW, Associate Professor of Medicine, Boston University School of Medicine

---

[1] Institute of Medicine forums and roundtables do not issue, review, or approve individual documents. The responsibility for the published workshop summary rests with the workshop rapporteur and the institution.

TERRI ANN PARNELL, Principal and Founder, Health Literacy Partners, LLC
KIM PARSON, Strategic Consultant, Proactive Care Strategies, Humana
KAVITA PATEL, Managing Director for Clinical Transformation and Delivery, The Brookings Institute
ANDREW PLEASANT, Senior Director for Health Literacy and Research, Canyon Ranch Institute
LINDSEY A. ROBINSON, Thirteenth District Trustee, American Dental Association
STACEY ROSEN, Associate Professor of Cardiology and Vice President, Women's Health, The Katz Institute for Women's Health, Hofstra North Shore–Long Island Jewish School of Medicine
RIMA RUDD, Senior Lecturer on Health Literacy, Education, and Policy, Harvard School of Public Health
STEVEN RUSH, Director, Health Literacy Innovations, UnitedHealth Group
PAUL M. SCHYVE, Senior Advisor, Healthcare Improvement, The Joint Commission
MICHAEL VILLAIRE, Chief Executive Officer, Institute for Healthcare Advancement
EARNESTINE WILLIS, Kellner Professor in Pediatrics, Medical College of Wisconsin
MICHAEL WOLF, Professor, Medicine and Learning Sciences, Associate Division Chief–Research Division of General Internal Medicine, Feinberg School of Medicine, Northwestern University
WINSTON WONG, Medical Director, Community Benefit, Disparities Improvement and Quality Initiatives, Kaiser Permanente

Consultant

RUTH PARKER, Professor of Medicine, Pediatrics, and Public Health, Emory University School of Medicine

IOM Staff

LYLA M. HERNANDEZ, Senior Program Officer
MELISSA FRENCH, Associate Program Officer
ANDREW LEMERISE, Research Associate
ANGELA MARTIN, Senior Program Assistant (through April 3, 2015)
EMILY VOLLBRECHT, Senior Program Assistant (April 6, 2015, to present)
ROSE MARIE MARTINEZ, Director, Board on Population Health and Public Health Practice

Reviewers

This workshop summary has been reviewed in draft form by individuals chosen for their diverse perspectives and technical expertise. The purpose of this independent review is to provide candid and critical comments that will assist the institution in making its published workshop summary as sound as possible and to ensure that the workshop summary meets institutional standards for objectivity, evidence, and responsiveness to the study charge. The review comments and draft manuscript remain confidential to protect the integrity of the process. We wish to thank the following individuals for their review of this workshop summary:

MATT KREUTER, The Brown School, Washington University in St. Louis
SYDNEE LOGAN, U.S. Food and Drug Administration
JOSUHA SEIDMAN, Avalere Health
DAVID C. TORRES, MAXIMUS

Although the reviewers listed above have provided many constructive comments and suggestions, they did not see the final draft of the workshop summary before its release. The review of this workshop summary was overseen by **Ned Calogne,** The Colorado Trust. He was responsible for making certain that an independent examination of this workshop summary was carried out in accordance with institutional procedures and that all review comments were carefully considered. Responsibility for the final content of this workshop summary rests entirely with the rapporteur and the institution.

Acknowledgments

We are grateful to the sponsors of the Institute of Medicine Roundtable on Health Literacy who made it possible to plan and conduct the workshop on health literacy and consumer-facing technology, which this report summarizes. Sponsors from the U.S. Department of Health and Human Services are the Agency for Healthcare Research and Quality, Health Resources and Services Administration, National Institutes of Health, and Office of Disease Prevention and Health Promotion. Nonfederal sponsorship was provided by the Aetna Foundation; Bristol-Myers Squibb; California Dental Association; East Bay Community Foundation (Kaiser Permanente); Eli Lilly and Company; Health Literacy Missouri; Health Literacy Partners; Humana; Institute for Healthcare Advancement; Merck & Co., Inc.; North Shore–Long Island Jewish Health System; and UnitedHealth Group.

The workshop presentations were extremely interesting and stimulating and we would like to thank each of the speakers for their time and effort. Speakers are Patricia Dykes, Read Holman, Dean Hovey, Elizabeth Jordan, Katherine Kim, Alex Krist, Lana Moriarty, Catina O'Leary, Alison Rein, Lygeia Ricciardi, Rebecca Schnall, and Winston Wong. Thanks also go to the excellent moderators Suzanne Bakken, Pamela Jeffries, and Bernard Rosof.

Contents

ACRONYMS AND ABBREVIATIONS   xvii

1   INTRODUCTION   1
Organization of the Summary, 2

2   CONSUMER-FACING TECHNOLOGY: WHAT IS IT AND WHAT ARE THE ISSUES?   5
Discussion, 11

3   HEALTH LITERATE DIGITAL DESIGN AND STRATEGIES   15
Design Specification for Apps: A Case Study, 16
The Federal Digital Strategy and Health Literacy, 21
Patient Portals, 24
Reactions to the Panel Presentations, 30
Discussion, 32

4   CATALYZING WIDESPREAD INFORMED ENGAGEMENT   43
Consumer-Generated Health Information: Provider "Readiness," Attitudes, and Skills, 43
Incentives for Consumer Engagement, 48
Building a Fabric of Trust: Ethical, Legal, and Social Issues in the Era of eHealth and Big Data, 50
Discussion, 54

5 HEALTH INFORMATION TECHNOLOGY AND SELECTED
    POPULATIONS   63
    Issues and Use in Native American Populations, 63
    Mobile Technologies for Pregnant Women and New Mothers, 68
    Lessons Learned from the Workshop on Digital Health Strategies,
        Health Disparities, and Health Equity, 71
    Discussion, 74

6 REFLECTIONS ON THE DAY   81

REFERENCES   89

APPENDIXES

A WORKSHOP AGENDA   93
B BIOGRAPHICAL SKETCHES OF WORKSHOP SPEAKERS   97

Box, Figures, and Table

BOX

1-1 Statement of Task, 3

FIGURES

2-1 Age-adjusted prevalence of obesity and diagnosed diabetes among U.S. adults ages 18 years or older, 8

3-1 An information systems research framework used to design an end-user focused app, 17
3-2 An example of the app user interface developed by the design panel participants and the first mock-up of the home page and sexually transmitted disease report created by the researchers, 20
3-3 The home screen and a sexually transmitted disease report from the final mock-up of an HIV prevention app, 21
3-4 An example of the MyPreventiveCare user-friendly patient portal and the page detailing the preventive care a particular female patient needs, 27

4-1 A patient-facing webpage from PROSPECT, 47

5-1 Words that represent traditional Native American values are a piece of culturally grounded evidence, 66

TABLE

3-1 The Results of the First of Two Design Sessions Prior to Developing an App for HIV Prevention Among High-Risk Men Who Have Sex with Men, 19

Acronyms and Abbreviations

ACP   American College of Physicians
AHRQ   Agency for Healthcare Research and Quality

CDC   Centers for Disease Control and Prevention
CHIP   Children's Health Insurance Program

EHR   electronic health record

FDA   U.S. Food and Drug Administration
FERPA   Family Educational Rights and Privacy Act

GPS   global positioning system

HHS   U.S. Department of Health and Human Services
HIPAA   Health Insurance Portability and Accountability Act
HITECH   Health Information Technology for Economic and Clinical Health
HRSA   Health Resources and Services Administration

IDEA   Innovation, Design, Entrepreneurship and Action Lab
IOM   Institute of Medicine

LIJ   Long Island Jewish

NCAI	National Congress of American Indians
NCI	National Cancer Institute
NIH	National Institutes of Health
NLM	National Library of Medicine
ONC	Office of the National Coordinator for Health Information Technology
PCORI	Patient-Centered Outcomes Research Institute
PROSPECT	Promoting Respect and Ongoing Safety through Patient-centeredness, Engagement, Communication, and Technology
WIC	Special Supplemental Nutrition Program for Women, Infants, and Children
USPSTF	U.S. Preventive Services Task Force
VA	U.S. Department of Veterans Affairs

1

Introduction[1]

The proliferation of consumer-facing technology and personal health information technology has grown steadily over the past decade, and has certainly exploded over the past several years. As Bernard Rosof, chief executive officer of the Quality in Healthcare Advisory Group, noted in his introductory remarks to the workshop, many people have embraced smartphones and wearable health-monitoring devices to track their fitness and personal health information. Providers have made it easier for patients and caregivers to access health records and communicate through online patient portals. However, he added, the large volume of health-related information that these devices can generate and input into a health record can also lead to an increased amount of confusion on the part of users and caregivers.

A recent opinion piece in *The New York Times* (Wachter, 2015) spoke of the productivity paradox of information technology and the lag between the adoption of technology and the realization of technology gains. This article cited the lack of user-centered design for most health care software as one reason for that paradox. It called for better collaboration between academic researchers and software developers, but it also asked what Rosof considered an important question: What would be an ideal future? The

---

[1] The planning committee's role was limited to planning the workshop, and this summary has been prepared by the workshop rapporteur as a factual summary of what occurred at the workshop. Statements, recommendations, and opinions expressed are those of individual presenters and participants, and are not necessarily endorsed or verified by the Institute of Medicine (IOM), nor should they be construed as reflecting any group consensus.

article's author answers that the ideal future will have a technology that physicians suddenly cannot live without. Rosof amended this slightly to include patients and the health care team on the list of those who cannot live without a particular technology.

The goal of this workshop was to explore health literate practices in health information technology and then provide and consider the ramifications of this rapidly growing field on the health literacy of users.[2] Box 1-1 describes the workshop Statement of Task.

ORGANIZATION OF THE SUMMARY

The workshop (see Appendix A for the agenda) was organized by an independent planning committee in accordance with the procedures of the National Academies of Sciences, Engineering, and Medicine. The planning committee's members were Suzanne Bakken, roundtable member and alumni professor of nursing and professor of biomedical informatics at the Columbia University School of Nursing; Gillian Christie, health innovation analyst at The Vitality Institute; Garth Graham, roundtable member and president of the Aetna Foundation; Linda Harris, roundtable member and director of the division of health communication and eHealth in the Office of Disease Prevention and Health Promotion at the U.S. Department of Health and Human Services (HHS); Pamela Jeffries, vice provost for digital initiatives at Johns Hopkins University; Andrew Pleasant, roundtable member and senior director for health literacy and research at the Canyon Ranch Institute; and Ted Vickey, founder and president of FitWell, Inc.

This publication summarizes the discussions that occurred throughout the workshop, highlighting the lessons presented, practical strategies, and the needs and opportunities for improving health literacy in consumer-facing technology. Chapter 2 provides an overview of consumer-facing technology and the issues involved in creating, deploying, and adopting such technologies. Chapter 3 discusses health literate digital design and some of the strategies for creating health literate apps and patient portals that the federal government and other health organizations are using. Chapter 4 recounts the wide-ranging presentations and discussions centering on ways of catalyzing widespread informed engagement of both consumers and health care professionals in the effort to develop and use health literate consumer-facing technologies. Chapter 5 describes some of the efforts underway to use consumer-facing technologies with selected populations of

---

[2] The workshop did not include information about issues regarding access to and use of digital technology by socioeconomic status nor did it include information about the objective value of consumer-generated data.

> **BOX 1-1**
> **Statement of Task**
>
> An ad hoc committee will plan and conduct a public workshop on health literacy, new technology, and health. The workshop will feature invited presentations and discussions. The topics may include health literacy and the use of technology (e.g., social media) to inform health decision making, sharing health information via technology, or examples of health literacy best practices as they apply to the use of technology for health decisions. The committee will define the specific topics to be addressed, develop the agenda, select and invite speakers and other participants, and moderate the discussions. An individually authored summary of the presentations and discussions at the workshop will be prepared by a designated rapporteur in accordance with institutional guidelines.

Americans as a means of reducing health disparities. Chapter 6 covers the roundtable's reflections on the lessons learned at this workshop.

In accordance with the policies of the Institute of Medicine (IOM), the workshop did not attempt to establish any conclusions or recommendations about needs and future directions, focusing instead on issues identified by the speakers and workshop participants. In addition, the organizing committee's role was limited to planning the workshop. The workshop summary has been prepared by the workshop rapporteur as a factual summary of what occurred at the workshop.

2

Consumer-Facing Technology: What Is It and What Are the Issues?[1]

The workshop opened with an overview presentation by Ted Vickey, founder and president of FitWell, Inc. He began his talk by recounting how his passion for digital health was born out of his experience as the executive director of the White House Athletic Center charged with helping to manage the health and fitness of the President and his staff. During this assignment, White House staff repeatedly requested that he travel with the President, but his answer was always that he could not because he needed to stay in Washington to help the entire staff, not just those who traveled with the President. "I needed to find a way to eliminate the four physical walls of our fitness center and to become virtual," Vickey explained. As his physical fitness consulting business grew, other clients approached him about managing distance facilities and this increased his interest in and passion for digital health tools.

Turning to the subject at hand, Vickey asked the following question: "Can consumer-facing digital health technology really help people live healthier lives?" Before answering this question, he noted the number of workshop attendees whom, like him, were wearing activity-tracking devices and commented that certain people fear using this technology. He also remarked that "this area is so new and in flux that here is a great opportunity and an even greater potential to leverage this technology to help people lead healthier lives."

---

[1] This section is based on the presentation by Ted Vickey, founder and president of FitWell, Inc., and the statements are not endorsed or verified by the IOM.

Vickey pointed out that academic research suggests that there are more than 200 definitions for consumer-facing digital health technology, including eHealth and mHealth, gamification of health, and big data. He considers consumer-facing digital health technology to focus on applications (apps), wearables, and websites. He discussed some examples, starting with Fooducate, an app that enables a smartphone user to scan a food product's barcode while shopping and to receive a health score for that item. This app can be useful for providing teachable moments that can lead to purchasing decisions when parents are shopping with their children. A fitness tracking app called Runkeeper, which he used as part of his Ph.D. research project, tracks time and distance for a run and enables the user to share these data with his or her social network. A similar app from Nike connects to Facebook and enables friends and family to remotely cheer and even provide voice encouragement to runners as they make progress.

Recently, Vickey began using the iHeadache app to track his migraine headaches, including symptoms and preceding events that may have triggered the migraine. "What I was able to do with this app was then go in and have a more educated discussion with my physician about the headaches," explained Vickey.

One wearable device that he highlighted is a tattoo that sticks to the upper arm and monitors glucose levels in real time for diabetic individuals. Another device, from a company called Fitlinxx, is a heart monitor that resembles a Band-Aid and is meant to replace a bulkier chest-strap heart rate monitor. This device, which is placed over the heart, transmits heart rate both to a mobile phone app and to exercise equipment so that the user can monitor his or her heart rate while exercising. Vickey also mentioned the recently released Apple Watch as being part fitness device, but pointed out that its $350 price point is one that many people will be unable to afford and that its complexity may be beyond the abilities of some potential users. "What can we do to help them?" he asked.

Informational websites such as WebMD and Doctor Google, as well as government websites, are becoming an important avenue for patients to get health-related information, Vickey said. Health-related websites include PatientsLikeMe, which provides a means for patients to share real-world health experiences and to help similar users to connect with organizations that focus on specific health conditions. "If I had a rare disease and lived in San Diego and there were others in Boston with similar symptoms, I could now have this interface for connecting," said Vickey. "I realize that some physicians, some health groups may be nervous about what this does to the quality of health care, but it's happening. So how can we be part of that solution?"

Vickey then quoted Unity Stoakes, co-founder of StartUp Health, to illustrate one of the paradoxes of consumer-facing technology. "Digital health innovation takes longer than you think and happens faster than you think at the same exact time," said Stoakes. His organization is aiming to address this paradox by helping 1,000 health start-ups to reimagine and transform health care over the next decade based on the belief that entrepreneurs have the collective power to build the future of health care. Vickey also noted that other start-up incubators across the country and around the world are coming together and trying to figure out how to create a better approach to health care.

Sharing some statistics about smartphone use, Vickey noted that smartphone users keep their device within arm's reach 91 percent of the time, a transformation he considers remarkable given that the iPhone was first released in 2007. "What I find interesting now is that the computing power in the smartphones that we all have is more powerful than the computer used to put a man on the moon," he said, "so can we use that technology to move our agenda forward?" He also noted that many more people now use fitness apps than belong to health clubs, a worrisome trend for the health and fitness industry. Even more alarming to that industry is the fact that 73 percent of app users say they are healthier today because of those apps. Other statistics Vickey cited included

- Sixty-nine percent of mobile health users think that tracking their health and fitness on their smartphone is more important than using it for social networking or online shopping;
- Forty-six percent say that tracking has changed their overall approach to maintaining their own health or the health of another, suggesting that people are now using smartphone apps to manage the care of family members;
- Forty percent of people who use tracking devices say that doing so has led them to ask a health professional new questions or to get a second opinion; and
- Thirty-four percent say that it has affected a decision about how to treat an illness or a condition.

"These stats are impressive, and the technology is persuasive, but how can we make the connection and leverage these advancements in technology to impact chronic disease and to improve health? Because the world suggests a different story," Vickey said.

That different story starts with the fact that obesity levels continue to rise across the country, as does the prevalence of diabetes (see Figure 2-1). An increasing number of Americans with chronic diseases now account for 84 percent of the nation's health care dollars and 99 percent of Medicare spending (Anderson, 2010), with projections suggesting that this situation is likely to worsen. Nearly half of the U.S. population suffers from one or

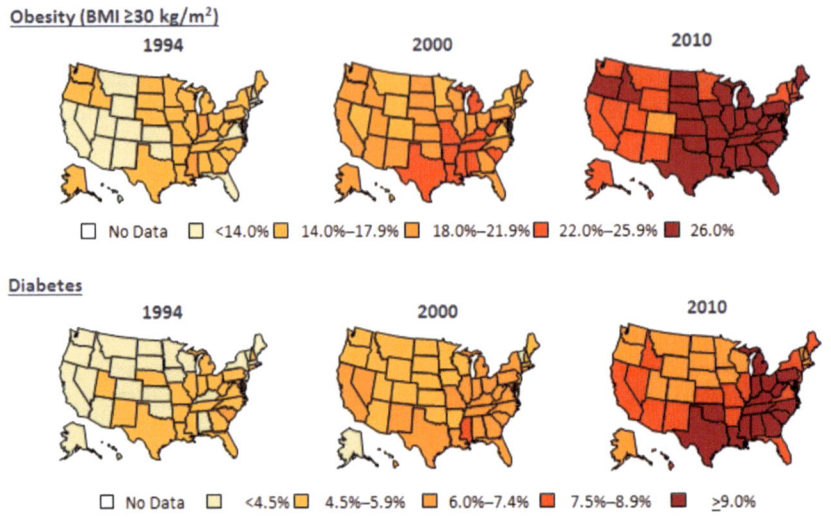

FIGURE 2-1 Age-adjusted prevalence of obesity and diagnosed diabetes among U.S. adults ages 18 years or older.
NOTE: BMI = body mass index.
SOURCE: Centers for Disease Control and Prevention's Division of Diabetes Translation. National Diabetes Surveillance System. http://www.cdc.gov/diabetes/statistics (accessed March 24, 2015). Vickey presentation, March 24, 2015.

more chronic diseases, and by 2020 the number of Americans suffering from multiple chronic diseases is expected to rise significantly (Bodenheimer et al., 2009), Vickey noted.

The other aspect of this different story is that while users report loving apps, health care professionals are still hesitant about using the data those apps generate. A recent survey, for example, found that 16 percent of health care providers are using mobile health apps in their own practices with their patients, and half of the health care providers surveyed expect to use these types of devices in their practice within the next 5 years. "So while the health care providers are well aware of the benefits, most are still reluctant to jump in, which begs the question of why," said Vickey. Consumers, he said, report that they are using these apps and devices to track their health goals, become aware of health issues, and become motivated. Regarding this last point, he said a major reason why people hire a personal trainer is for motivation and accountability. He also mentioned that he has a scale at home that not only reports his weight via the Internet to his physician via his electronic health record (EHR), but it also Tweets his weight to his followers, which makes him accountable to a large group of people. "That's where we can leverage this technology," he said.

The *Pew Mobile Health Report* (Fox and Duggan, 2012) suggests there are many different groups that use smartphones to gather health information, particularly Latinos and African Americans ages 18 to 49, and those with college degrees. To be specific, though, Vickey spoke about his father as someone who has a smartphone and could benefit from the health information it could collect, yet has trouble typing on his smartphone and loses connection to the Internet when he leaves his house. "Is there a way that we can help him manage his high blood pressure and the medications he takes?" asked Vickey. "I think the answer is yes." To illustrate that point, he recounted an experience he had in the Bronx, the poorest U.S. congressional district, when he was speaking with a nutritionist about what she was doing with the community to improve eating habits there. Given the widespread use of smartphones by people living in that community, he expected that she would teach residents to use the smartphone as a readily available means of keeping a food journal. That would be too complicated, she said, so Vickey suggested having her clients use their phones' camera function to create a picture album of the foods they were preparing and eating. That idea appealed to the nutritionist and is being tested.

Investments in consumer-facing health information technologies continues to rise, he then noted, increasing from $1 billion in 2011 to $4.6 billion in 2014. UnderArmour, for example, just acquired makers of two of the more popular mobile fitness apps: MyFitnessPal for $450 million and Endomondo for another $85 million. These two apps combined have a user base of 120 million people, compared to the fitness industry with 58 million health club members. They provide examples of how the convergence of technology and health care is helping to change how consumers get health care information and use it to change their behaviors. Four out of five Americans now own a smartphone and are using it more and more on a daily basis, said Vickey. Moreover, smartphone users are becoming more technically savvy, particularly seniors who want to use technology to access information about their health care. For example, more than two-thirds of seniors prefer to use self-care technology to independently manage their health, and more than 60 percent are willing to wear a health-monitoring device to track vital signs, such as heart rate and blood pressure. Sixty percent of seniors are somewhat or very likely to turn to online communities for health information, and one-quarter of them now regularly use their smartphones for managing their health, a figure that is expected to grow to 42 percent over the next 5 years as the number, variety, and utility of consumer-facing tools increases, Vickey said.

Researchers from the Pew Research Center have talked about peer-to-peer health care, when the Internet is giving patients and caregivers access to both information and each other, creating a forum of sorts where patients can talk about their ailments and treatments. Vickey believes the clear intentions of Apple, Google, and Microsoft to move into the digital health space is a good thing, though not everyone agrees with this sentiment. Apple, for example, has released a research kit that allows researchers to collect information easily and even recruit people for clinical trials. He said that within a day of announcing that there was a Parkinson's disease research kit, some 10,000 people applied to be part of a clinical trial. "How many researchers would love to have that sample set of 10,000 people?" asked Vickey.

Development of these kinds of tools presents challenges. Privacy and data ownership are two issues that need to be addressed. For example, Vickey conducted a research project in which he collected more than 7 million Tweets in which people shared their running workout routines for more than 1 year. From some of these Tweets he could find out a person's routine, the distance run, time and heart rate, and any music listened to during exercise. He could also identify an individual's running routes and the time of day that person ran, which may not be ideal information to share. "We need to help educate developers and users about what is being shared," said Vickey. Another challenge arises from a lack of standards. Last year, he noted, the IOM issued a discussion paper on designing health literate mobile apps (Broderick et al., 2014).

The London School of Economics has created an app called Mappiness that occasionally asks smartphone users how happy they are feeling and where they are at a particular moment, which enables the developers to monitor in real time how people across the United Kingdom are feeling. Mappiness, then, is a tool for monitoring one aspect of well-being on a national level, and it enables a new sort of measurement that was not possible before. As management expert Peter Drucker said, "You can't manage what you can't measure."

Vickey then presented additional examples of what could be considered boundary-pushing consumer-facing technology. GoBe is a combination wrist-worn sensor and a smartphone app that measures, through the skin, calorie intake, nutritional intake, and calories burned. Whether this claim is accurate or not (Vickey said he believes it is not), this wearable's developers raised $1 million through the crowdfunding site Indiegogo because as Vickey put it, people want this type of technology to work.

Another smartphone app called PlushCare enables "face-to-face" appointments with a physician—but only in California because current law does not allow a physician in one state to treat patients in another state. The U.S. Food and Drug Administration (FDA) and Congress are aware of this issue and are working on a solution, Vickey said. "But sometimes, innovation in digital health is faster than what we are used to and the regulatory path is still a little confusing."

Concluding his remarks, Vickey called digital health a most interesting space for health literacy. "This area of technology is rapidly growing and changing, but there remain problems with access and equity. There seems to be real potential here to make a difference in the lives of people, lots and lots of people, so that they can live healthier lives, but this technology still remains unproven and the lack of scientific proof puts sustained growth of this consumer-facing health technology at some sort of risk. People will ask if this is just another fad," Vickey said, adding that he hoped this workshop would start a discussion about how health literacy can help create sustained behavior change in people's lives through these technologies.

DISCUSSION

During the brief discussion period following this presentation, Bernard Rosof asked Vickey what he thought consumer-facing technology would look like over the next 10 to 15 years and what effects it will have on health, chronic disease, and improvement of health in general. Vickey responded that he believes the field is at a great place today. "I've been in the health and fitness industry for 20 years, and I've never been as excited as I am today about the potential of where we're going," he said. Apps, wearables, and websites are getting easier to use, which is a positive, but he fears that without good science behind them, they will not enable behavior change. "That's why I think the next step is coming together, creating a set of standards, and creating opportunities to bring Apple, Google, and Microsoft to the table so they can be part of the solution," he said.

Michael Paasche-Orlow, associate professor of medicine at the Boston University School of Medicine, voiced his concern that these technologies will drive an increase in disparities because the most avid users are the "wealthy, worried, and well," as he put it. He asked Vickey if had any ideas on how to address this situation. Vickey agreed that this was indeed a problem and one of his main concerns as well. "The people that need the technology may not be using the technology because they can't afford it." However, tracker devices, for example, are now available for less than $20, and it may be possible to capitalize on the fact that smartphone use seems to span all socioeconomic levels so they can be used as health-monitoring devices. Rosof commented that while the literature supports the notion that smartphones are becoming ubiquitous in American society, the issue may be one of health literacy and the transfer of appropriate information rather than whether someone can acquire a smartphone. Terry Davis, professor of medicine and pediatrics at the Louisiana State University Health Sciences Center, added that in her research with new mothers coming into a very low-income clinic, all of the women had smartphones and all had downloaded an app for pregnant mothers that provided a wealth of information on what they should do during pregnancy to have a healthy baby. Her concern, though, was that many of these women had low literacy, and she wondered if they were able to use the information in those apps.

Laurie Francis, senior director of clinical operations and quality at the Oregon Primary Care Association, agreed that the problem was not so much about the affordability of a smartphone, but the fact that apps need to speak to where people are in their lives rather than where they need to be with regard to their health. "Controlling A1C when you're working three jobs or trying to get shoes for your kids or living on the street is not your top priority," she said. "So how do we build apps that are respectful and connecting?" Regarding the latter, she wondered if apps can eliminate the provider team from the behavior change equation given that the behavior change needed to overcome many chronic diseases often has little to do with the physician or care team. "We always turn to the doctor to help us with chronic care, which is often not generated by a lack of medical care, but a history of many challenges," said Francis. Vickey noted that consumer-facing technology can play an important role without the involvement of the physician and that it can also help connect individuals with others who can help them, such as the nutritionist, personal trainer, mental health specialist, and other members of a wellness team. The key to realizing this potential, he added, is to involve the user in these discussions. "We need to understand what they want and how they want it and bring them to the table and say 'help us design these apps and these wearable devices,'" he said.

Jennifer Dillaha, medical director for immunizations and medical advisor for health literacy and communication at the Arkansas Department of Health, noted that this presentation helped her think of a connection that might offer a way to help overcome learned helplessness, which often plagues those with chronic illnesses who seem unable to make the necessary changes to improve their health (Seligman, 2012). "When you were talking it made me wonder if some of these apps could be used in such a way as to help people who don't believe they can have control or make a change to overcome that sense of learned helplessness and manage their current conditions," she said. Vickey agreed that apps could help with that aspect of managing chronic disease, but his main concern is that there are tens of thousands of apps and no good way for the average person to pick those that provide good information. "People can create apps and then can claim to be health experts or health literacy experts, but they may not be," said Vickey. He hopes that someday there will be a stamp of approval for apps as well as a means to measure the effectiveness of apps at changing health behavior.

Rosof remarked that this last comment seemed to be a call for standardization, and Vickey said it was. "This is the new version of snake oil salesman, and we need to have those standards," he noted. The question is who will create the standards, and he wondered if the roundtable could play a role by creating the momentum needed to bring together the appropriate stakeholders to establish standards. Workshop participant Robert Logan, communications research scientist at the National Library of Medicine (NLM), commented that in his role as a federal official, standards mean FDA. "Do you really want FDA to take charge of this? What about having the industry itself take charge of this?" he asked. He said he doubted that the broadcast industry, if it had to do it all over again, would have asked the government to create the Federal Communications Commission to end the confusion that reigned over airwave rights, and he implored this community to think hard before asking a federal agency to get involved in creating standards.

Christopher Dezii, director of Healthcare Quality and Performance Measures at Bristol-Myers Squibb, wondered if the field should start working on interoperability with respect to the feedback that consumer-facing technology can provide to physicians. Vickey agreed and said there needs to be a discussion about how to create interoperability that does not dictate actions, but rather provides feedback and advice. "I was reading an article a couple of months ago that said these technologies won't work until they tell us what to do, and I don't think I want a technology to tell me what to do," he said.

Winston Wong, medical director for community benefit disparities improvement and quality initiatives at Kaiser Permanente, asked if consumer-facing health technology can facilitate public health, citing the recent outbreak of measles as a public health failure and wondering if an app or other health technology could facilitate the advancement of public health in a health literate manner. Vickey responded that software is already being used to track influenza outbreaks by monitoring Twitter posts in which people tweet about their symptoms. "This technology is opening up with so many new ways of looking at things that we may not have done before," said Vickey. "I go back to the Mappiness example that sends out push notifications to find out where people are and how they feel. Can we do the same thing when it comes to health? I think we can, and while we don't have all the answers now, I think by having organizations such as the IOM and others bring together all of the stakeholders to the table to find consensus, that we can find a way to do that."

Rosof added that he is working on a program with the American College of Physicians (ACP) called I Raise the Rates that aims to increase the rates of immunization. "I think that it requires more than an iPhone or something digital, it requires an education process around that," he said, adding that champions, in addition to social media, are needed to encourage public education about these issues.

Michael Villaire, chief executive officer of the Institute for Healthcare Advancement, worries that these devices and apps might be disempowering in the long run, citing the food score app that Vickey described in his talk. "That's a great tool, but when it replaces our own ability to look at food and make a choice, is that a good thing?" What happens, he said, when a person is in the grocery store without his or her smartphone and cannot access food information? "How are we able to make those decisions if we've been relying on the app to make those decisions for us?" he asked. Another problem, added Vickey, is what to do with all of the information that these technologies generate. His FitBit, for example, has recorded more than 7 million steps since he started wearing it. "So what?" he said. "I think what happens now is that a lot of these data are in a data silo. So I have my step information here, I have my blood pressure information here, I have my food journaling here. But what I'm seeing now in the industry is finally some interoperability of people coming together and being able to see that information as one."

Vickey commented that consumer-facing technologies may eventually serve as a diagnostic tool for physicians in much the same way that a modern car's onboard computer provides diagnostic information for an auto mechanic. He noted that he is working on a project with a San Diego middle school that will outfit everyone with a FitBit to monitor heart rates when the students take tests and to monitor how well they sleep the night before a test. The goal is to use the resulting data as part of a wellness program.

Alicia Fernandez, professor of clinical medicine at the University of California, San Francisco, commented that most of her primary care patients are poorly educated and have a hard time learning how to use even a simple pedometer, let alone a FitBit. Many have a smartphone, but have no idea how to download an app, she said. She wondered if there was some new position—a medical assistant informatician or a pharmacist informatician—whose job could be to help patients download apps and set them up, then teach patients how to use these new technologies in much the same way that she has someone on her staff who reviews medication information with a patient. "I think you just created a new job that I would love to have," said Vickey in response to her suggestion. He noted that he has been advising health clubs, fitness centers, and personal trainers to offer people who get a FitBit or other device to bring it to the club for help setting it up. "I think that there's an opportunity to be able to have someone in a doctor's office, in a health club, in a Walgreens to be able to download these apps and educate people on the wearables," said Vickey in concluding the discussion period.

3

Health Literate Digital Design and Strategies

The workshop's first panel session featured three presentations, then reactions to those presentations by representatives of the entrepreneurial private sector, the foundation world, and government. Rebecca Schnall, assistant professor of nursing at the Columbia University School of Nursing, described the use of rigorous, user-centered design methods to understand the needs of a mobile app for HIV prevention among high-risk men who have sex with men. Read Holman, program director and senior advisor on internal entrepreneurship at the HHS Innovation, Design, Entrepreneurship and Action (IDEA) Lab in the Office of the Chief Technology Officer at HHS, discussed the federal government's digital strategy as a framework for spurring health literacy. Alex Krist, associate professor of family medicine and population health at Virginia Commonwealth University, spoke about patient portals as an example of a consumer-facing health technology. The three experts who commented on these presentations were Dean Hovey, an experienced entrepreneur and currently president and chief executive officer of Digifit; Catina O'Leary, president and chief executive officer of Health Literacy Missouri; and Lana Moriarty, director of the Office of the National Coordinator for Health Information Technology's (ONC's) Office of Consumer eHealth. An open discussion moderated by Susan Bakken, alumni professor of nursing and professor of biomedical informatics at Columbia University School of Nursing, and Bernard Rosof, followed the presentations and reactions.

DESIGN SPECIFICATION FOR APPS: A CASE STUDY[1]

To begin her presentation, Schnall said she was going to highlight a different approach to app design, one that involved speaking to end users and thinking about behavior change before starting the design process. This approach, she said, contrasts with the way most health-related apps have been designed, which is to create the app, put it into the app store, and then see if it gets used and helps change behavior. She noted that while mobile health technology has the potential to change health-related behaviors, there is little research evidence to date to support how these technologies can change health behaviors and outcomes in a meaningful way over the long term. She also pointed out that current estimates show some 40,000 apps are available that focus specifically on health-related activities and outcomes.

The goal of her group's work, which was funded by the Centers for Disease Control and Prevention (CDC), was to use rigorous, user-centered design methods to understand what features were most needed in a mobile app for HIV prevention aimed at high-risk men who have sex with men. This population continues to experience an increase in the number of new HIV infections, particularly in young Latino and African American men, despite the fact that the number of new cases in the American population in general has remained constant over the past few years. "We need something to target this population," said Schnall, and given the age of the target population, mobile health technology in the form of an app should be an appropriate venue for delivering health information. "Many of our participants were in low socioeconomic groups, but even though they're not really sure where they're getting their next lunch or where they're going to sleep tonight, they all have a smartphone," she explained.

The design framework she and her colleagues used is based on design science, a systematic form of designing with three iterative cycles: a relevance cycle, a design cycle, and a rigor cycle (see Figure 3-1). Not many of the 40,000 available mobile health apps or health information technology systems that are built today take all of these of these areas into consideration, Schnall explained, and some do not consider any of these aspects in their design. To identify the environmental factors that they needed to consider when designing this app, Schnall and her colleagues conducted focus groups with potential end users. They then looked at the existing knowledge base and identified what methods had already been used and tested for HIV prevention in terms of mobile health applications. They also

---

[1] This section is based on the presentation by Rebecca Schnall, assistant professor of nursing at the Columbia University School of Nursing, and the statements are not endorsed or verified by the IOM.

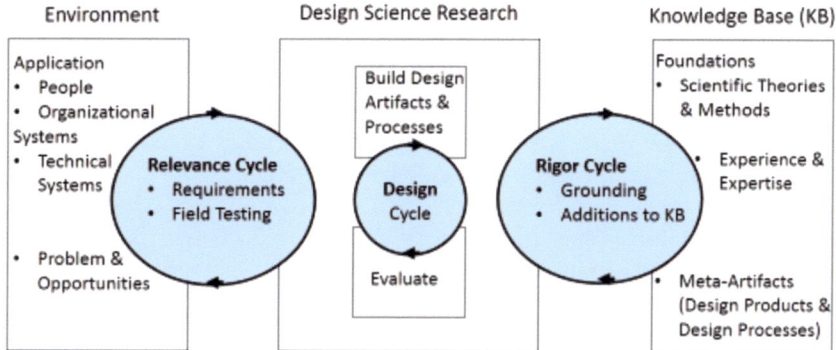

FIGURE 3-1 An information systems research framework used to design an end-user-focused app.
SOURCE: Schnall presentation, March 24, 2015.

considered how to test the app so they could determine how end users were able to use it and whether it was effective at changing behavior.

Going into more detail, Schnall explained that she and her colleagues conducted a series of 5 focus groups involving 33 high-risk men who have sex with men of ages ranging from 13 to 64. The focus groups included whites, African Americans, and Latinos, with one group consisting of only Spanish speakers. The results, said Schnall in response to a question, were largely congruent among the groups. A thematic analysis of the focus group sessions revealed five broad categories of what the participants wanted in an app:

- Information management, or the ability to manage their own health information, such as the time of their most recent HIV test or physical;
- How to stay healthy, including information on diet and exercise;
- HIV testing information;
- Chat or other communication functions that would enable them to stay in contact with peers, health counselors, and health care providers; and
- Access to resources.

With the relevance cycle complete, Schnall's team conducted activities related to the rigor cycle, which included an environmental scan of the existing literature related to both mobile health interventions and electronic health interventions that had been used with high-risk men who have sex with men to target HIV prevention behaviors. One goal of this literature review, which included both the peer-reviewed and grey literature (Schnall et al., 2014), was to find out about existing apps and the degree to which any of them had been studied. "Of the studies that we did include in our systematic review, there have been no rigorous studies of mobile health interventions in the study population," said Schnall.

The final cycle, the design cycle, had two components: the develop/build and evaluation phases, with activities centered on creating a highly usable app that incorporated the five categories of what users wanted in an app. As part of the design phase, Schnall and her colleagues conducted two 90-minute design sessions with the same group of 6 participants, ages 20 to 25, who were asked to tell the developers what the app should look like given the 5 broad categories. As an example of the responses in the first design session (see Table 3-1), the participants said they wanted a log of past partners to be part of the information management category so that if they tested positive for HIV at a later date, they could communicate with past partners if they so desired.

With regard to HIV testing, the participants had novel and innovative suggestions of the things they needed, said Schnall. "They all know that you need to get tested for HIV, but they had deeper health information needs as well as functionality for their app that were things we hadn't thought of ourselves as researchers," she said. For example, the participants said they not only want HIV testing site information, they wanted a global positioning system (GPS) location on how to get to the site, other users' rating of the site, and wait times at that site. They also wanted information on the difference between anonymous and confidential testing.

Following that first design session, at which all of the discussions were recorded, the researchers coded a first iteration of the app. They then held the second design session to get input from the participants on the user interface. Over a 2-hour session, the participants discussed what they wanted the app to look and feel like. After reviewing existing apps and splitting into two groups of three, the participants drew pictures of what the app user interface should look like (see Figure 3-2) and the researchers created mock-ups using PowerPoint for comment by the participants.

Next, the researchers conducted two types of usability assessments, both heuristic evaluation and end-user usability testing, on one of the mock-ups. Heuristic evaluation was conducted with informaticians and others who have expertise in user interface, design, usability principles, errors, and other important factors. End-user usability testing was conducted with high-risk men who have sex with men who were also given use cases to guide them in testing the mock-ups. Based on the heuristic evaluations, the researchers made 112 changes to the mock-up over 5 iterations, while end-user usability testing led to 55 more changes. Schnall said

TABLE 3-1 The Results of the First of Two Design Sessions Prior to Developing an App for HIV Prevention Among High-Risk Men Who Have Sex with Men

Topic Area	What	How
My Information Management	Log of Past Partners	Date, HIV Status, Rating of Experience
Staying Healthy	HIV Information	Videos
		Current Scams
	Prevention	HIV Risk Assessment Tool
		Updates on Pre-Exposure (PrEP) Studies
		Condom Size and Type Selector
	Diet/Fitness	Body Mass Index Calculator
		Exercise Tracker
HIV Testing	HIV Testing Site Info	Global Positioning System (GPS) Location
		Rating
		Cost
		Waiting Time
	Testing Log	Picture of Test Results
		Last Date Tested
Chat/Communication	Medical Providers	Contact for PrEP
		Link to Emergency Contact/Resources
		Live Hotline
	Social/Peer	Forums for Social Support
		Social Media Links
Resources	Support Group Locations	Voice Activated "Siri"
		GPS Mapping
	Condom Distribution Locations	GPS Mapping and Information on Condom Distribution Sites
	Latest HIV News	Newsfeeds

SOURCE: Schnall presentation, March 24, 2015.

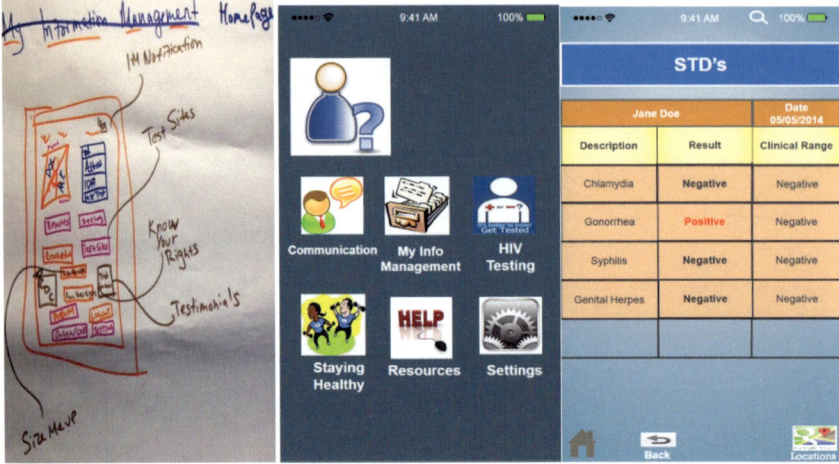

FIGURE 3-2 An example of the app user interface developed by the design panel participants and the first mock-up of the home page and sexually transmitted disease report created by the researchers.
SOURCE: Schnall presentation, March 24, 2015.

it was important that not all of the end users they recruited for usability testing were smartphone users, as each type of user provided valuable input that went into the final mock-up (see Figure 3-3). She also noted that the sexually transmitted disease report screen underwent the most remarkable changes, both in terms of the overall look of the page and the use of colors to denote the difference between a positive and a negative test result.

In closing, Schnall stressed the importance of making the design process iterative and of including input from end users about their needs. "We had our research team that was commenting and analyzing as we went through all this design process, but we also included our end users at every stage of the process in thinking about what our end product would be," she said. In the end, the synthesis of end-user feedback with content expert advice provided the foundation for the development of a highly usable and useful app. In response to a question, Schnall added that she plans to build this app for both English and Spanish speakers and that she did not think that content in the two versions would differ much.

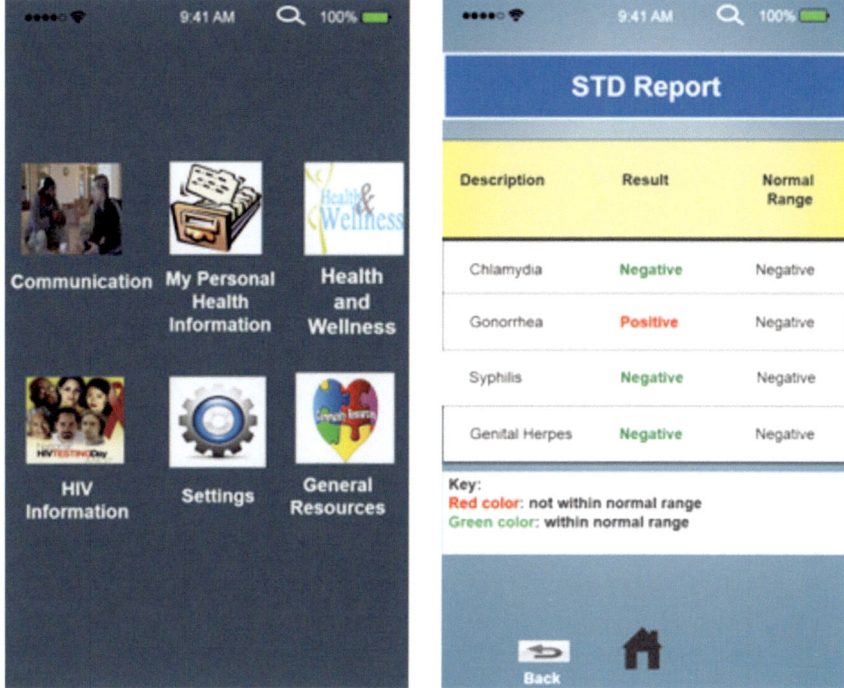

FIGURE 3-3 The home screen and a sexually transmitted disease (STD) report from the final mock-up of an HIV prevention app.
SOURCE: Schnall presentation, March 24, 2015.

THE FEDERAL DIGITAL STRATEGY AND HEALTH LITERACY[2]

Read Holman began his presentation by explaining that part of his role at HHS is to bring what he called "entrepreneurial methodologies" of the sort that are often associated with Silicon Valley into HHS. One of these entrepreneurial methodologies is known as lean start-up, which he said is fundamentally the principles of the scientific method brought to design. "It's do we know what we are building is actually working," he said. "How do we gather evidence, to build on the shoulders of giants if you will, but our giants just happen to be our end users?"

He then shared a brief anecdote to illustrate what he considers a good example of easy-to-use consumer-facing technology. While preparing his

---

[2] This section is based on the presentation by Read Holman, program director and senior advisor on internal entrepreneurship at the HHS IDEA Lab in the Office of the Chief Technology Officer at HHS, and the statements are not endorsed or verified by the IOM.

slides for this presentation, he struggled with what should have been a simple task of inserting page numbers onto each slide. Using the software's help function got him nowhere, so like many others, he used Google to search for an answer. It appeared immediately without the need to even click on a link or scroll anywhere. What struck him about the ease with which Google provided him with an answer is that people do this every day for health-related questions. Intrigued, he typed "What is Huntington's disease?" into the Google search box and again, the answer appeared. "I didn't have to click on anything, I didn't have to dive in through any website," said Holman. "This is the consumer-facing technology that we're all talking about."

Turning to the subject of the federal digital strategy and how it applies to health literacy, Holman said developers of the strategy did not have health literacy in mind. Instead, the strategy was aimed at the larger world of digital government and the direction of the information technology industry and its impact on society. The document that lays out the federal digital strategy (The White House, 2012) breaks out four strategic principles:

1. It should be information-centric, which focuses on the need for government to decouple the data and information layer from the presentation layer;
2. It should have a shared platform, which focuses on the need for government to work better with itself;
3. It should be customer-centric, that is, customers should be able to get their content anytime, anywhere, and on any device; and
4. It must have strengthened security and privacy processes.

Going into more detail about the first principle, that data and presentation should be separate considerations, Holman showed a data-dense, difficult-to-read spreadsheet of all the hospitals in the United States that accept Medicare patients and called that data. He then showed two of the many ways of visualizing those data to illustrate the difference between data and presentation. By separating data from presentation, the digital strategy creates an important framework for creating and displaying information in a way that is centered on the user, not the data generator. This framework consists of the presentation and data layers plus a management layer that sits between the two and provides the mechanisms by which users can get into the data, the way in which the data are released, and then how the data get converted into a suitable presentation format. Each of these layers, said Holman, exists in its own world. Addressing each component separately allows for achieving the ultimate goal, which is to create a better experience for users and provide better service to the American people. He noted that in the presentation layer, both the government and the private sector have roles to play in getting information from the government to the public.

The goal of creating this framework is to make data, whether they are numbers or words in a structured format, useful to the American people. With regard to the management layer, the goal is to provide easy access to the data through the development of application program interfaces and data formats while addressing concerns about privacy and security, Holman explained. The goal of the presentation layer is to provide excellent customer service and a great user experience. The latter is important, he noted, because the purpose of having a coherent digital strategy is to influence behavior. "Providing a useful and beautiful website is pointless if nobody is going to the website, or you're not having an impact on their lives," he said.

The federal government has many websites and most are "pretty ugly," Holman said in acknowledging that the private sector is better at designing a great experience for consumers. Recognizing that fact, the federal government is focusing on the data and management layer. As an example, he referred the workshop audience to the website healthdata.gov, which is where the federal government makes available more than 17,000 datasets related to health. This is not a site aimed at the American consumer, but rather those who want to create content and make information available to their customers.

Another example Holman discussed involved content syndication, the notion that content can be created once and then published by others on their own websites. CDC, for instance, prepares a wide range of Web-based information that is designed for publication on both private sector and government agency websites in a way that best meets the needs of those content providers through their ability to adjust the presentation layer. Holman also highlighted the "Blue Button" initiative, which is intended to allow every American to go online and download his or her health records and use that information for health improvement (Turvey et al., 2014).

In focusing on the data and management levels, the government aims to support the private sector in meaningful ways, such as by providing guidance and standards and by publishing research. As part of this effort, the government has created a set of challenges and prizes as a means of providing incentives to the private sector to develop new ways of presenting information to the American public. These challenges, authorized as part of the America Competes Act, have spurred competition in the private sector to create novel user experiences from the data that the government makes available. One challenge, for example, was to create an attractive patient record that an individual can download using the Blue Button. More than 230 developers responded, producing what Holman characterized as a number of beautiful and inspiring examples of apps and websites for displaying patient records.

Holman explained that while the government is publishing standards and guidance to help the private sector, and is largely leaving presentation-layer development to the private sector, it will jump in when the private sector is not succeeding in a particular area. In those cases, the government uses best practices from the literature and the start-up world and focuses on using iterative design methodologies that involve interacting with customers and patients. In the best cases, the iterations are small and the process grows a presentation format in collaboration with the end user. When this process is done using the scientific method, said Holman, the outcome will be a good-looking, usable, and useful product that serves the American people and drives behavior. He noted that government websites are increasingly being built using this approach to responsive design to produce websites, mobile apps, and tablet apps that are consistent in the way they present information.

In what he called a quick note about a data-driven future, Holman quoted President Obama, who said, "We want every American ultimately to be able to securely access and analyze their own health data so that they can make the best decisions for themselves and for their families." Meeting this goal will be difficult without health literate, consumer-facing technologies, for most Americans are not going to download their entire patient record, create macros in Excel, and analyze their data. Instead, consumers will rely on presentation layers such as the Google search page and Apple's Siri interface to create a user-friendly, usable experience. He commented that asking Siri the question "What is Huntington's disease?" produces the Wikipedia entry, but other queries, such as "How many calories have I burned?" produce fewer satisfying responses today. The question, said Holman, is "How can we get to that place where the one consumer-facing technology is that personal digital assistant?" The answer, he added, is near. In closing, he noted that the only way to ensure that the right data and the right information are getting to the consumer is to turn to the data layer and to ensure that the data are structured in a way that massive algorithms and search engines can digest them and present them to the user in a manner that is both informative and that changes behavior.

PATIENT PORTALS[3]

Alex Krist, who is both a practicing family physician and researcher, has been trying over the past decade to make patient portals more patient centered and to create an experience for patients that enables them to both

---

[3] This section is based on the presentation by Alex Krist, associate professor of family medicine and population health at Virginia Commonwealth University, and the statements are not endorsed or verified by the IOM.

access their health information and get advice based on that information about what they need to do to stay healthy. He noted before proceeding that he is a member of the U.S. Preventive Services Task Force (USPSTF), but that he would be talking about the work that he and his colleagues in Oregon, at the University of New Mexico, at Virginia Commonwealth University, and in the Office of Health Promotion and Disease Prevention have been doing, and not as a representative of the task force.

When thinking about patient portals, one fact to keep in mind is that two-thirds of primary care practices now use EHRs and 60 percent are participating in meaningful use, which means that they need patient portals. What this means for patients, explained Krist, is that they might have distinct portals with their primary care doctor, their specialists, the radiologist, the insurance company, and the laboratory company. He noted, in fact, that he had to register his daughter for a portal for an outpatient surgery center before she had surgery. The availability of so many portals, each with its own design, can create a situation that is challenging for patients to negotiate. At the same time, patients want to do many tasks with their portals, such as examining their EHRs to make sure they are correct, tracking expenses, avoiding duplicate tests, keeping their doctors informed of what is going on with their health, managing their families' health status, getting treatments that are tailored to them personally, and managing their health and lifestyle. Moreover, they want to be able to move from doctor to doctor, care setting to care setting, and take all of this information with them.

What portals are actually doing for patients is another matter, said Krist. To a large extent, he said, they function simply as a window to look at a patient's physician record, and those records are written in doctor language. "It's hard for doctors to understand what's in that information and unreasonable to expect patients to understand that information," said Krist. So while patients can see their lists of diagnoses, medicines, allergies, test results, and the like, and sometimes even doctors' notes, patients are often limited in what they can then do with this information. Laboratory results, for example, are often accompanied by reference ranges that do not apply to all patients and usually refer to worst case scenarios.

In addition, guidelines are becoming increasingly complex, making it difficult for patients to know what to do to improve their health even with the information in their health record. For example, the USPSTF makes a recommendation on the use of aspirin to prevent heart attacks, and this guideline says that a man age 45 to 79 should take aspirin if the benefit of preventing a heart attack outweighs the risk of gastrointestinal bleeding that can result from aspirin therapy. "That's tremendously difficult for a doctor to interpret, let alone a patient to interpret, who wants to know should I take an aspirin or should I not take an aspirin," said Krist. To be fair, he added, these USPSTF guidelines are meant for clinicians, not patients. He also noted that the task force is creating consumer-directed guides and that doctors' portals are trying to help patients make sense of these guidelines, though often physicians need to configure alerts, such as when their patients are overdue for immunizations.

Krist and his colleagues have been struggling with how to help patients truly understand the preventive care they need to stay healthy and to take action on that information. Their quest to solve those problems began with a series of grants that started in 2007 and has benefited from collaboration with the healthfinder.gov staff. The healthfinder.gov website was created with a user-centered design approach that includes formative and usability testing involving more than 700 patients, some of whom were of low literacy. It is also evidence based and the patient can tailor the site based on age and gender. As an example, Krist said that a woman can enter that she is pregnant. In turn she will receive a list of all of the preventing services that are covered by the Patient Protection and Affordable Care Act and that the USPSTF and other groups recommend. This design is based on the Health Literate Care model, Krist explained, and takes a universal precautions approach that assumes that everyone is at risk for not understanding the information. Even with taking a universal precautions approach, he noted, patients can take away different meanings than what health care professionals intend.

Taking this approach one step further, Krist's team is attempting to link into doctors' EHRs, make sense of the data there, apply national guidelines, and generate concrete advice in patient-centered terms that are specific for each individual. The result is MyPreventiveCare, which aims to translate into lay language all of the information in guidelines as applied to the information in each patient's EHR. This is done using an application that is embedded into patient portals and that takes the content of a patient's EHR, applies clinical information to that content, and produces advice in a user-friendly form that can go from prevention to disease management, with links to additional information on each piece of advice (see Figure 3-4). "I often liken it to the doctor sitting next to the patient and saying here are the things I want you to look at and go over, and it's personalized based on their profile," said Krist. The design and functionality are modeled after healthfinder.gov and it is tailored to meet patient preferences and to integrate into the typical workflow of primary care.

Referring to the first two presentations in this session, Krist reiterated the importance of getting stakeholder input during the design process. "Throughout the whole process we have patient and clinician advisory boards that are influencing our design iteratively. We have had hundreds of practiced learning collaboratives where clinicians are talking about how they want to use this information, what's important for their patients, and how they want to integrate it into the workflow," he explained. "We have

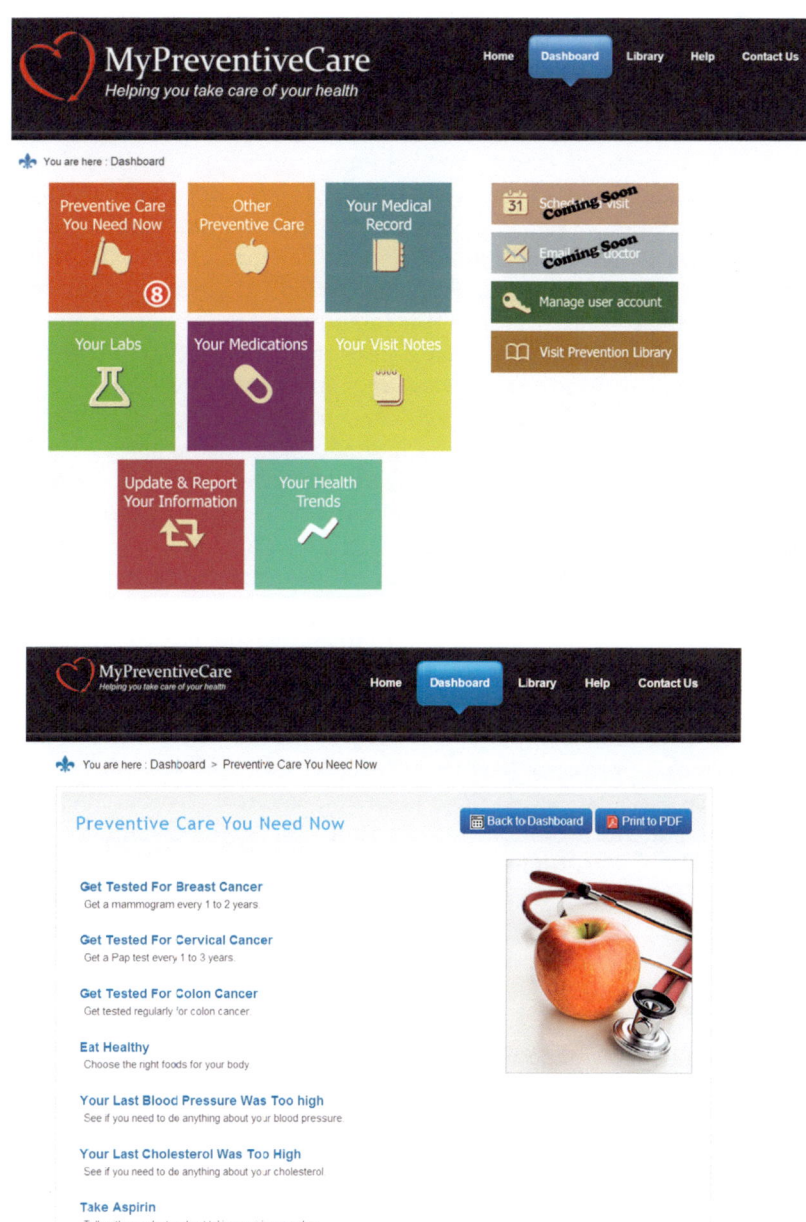

FIGURE 3-4 An example of the MyPreventiveCare user-friendly patient portal and the page detailing the preventive care a particular female patient needs.
SOURCE: Krist presentation, March 24, 2015.

diaries where clinicians, nurses, and other staff can enter their experiences with how this is going. We do usability testing, and then we have open comments for patients using the system to give us feedback whenever they like."

Krist and his collaborators have conducted randomized, controlled clinical trials to test whether tailored information improves the delivery of recommended preventive services. They have also been able to study whether primary care practices can implement and use this portal and get their patients to use it. A recent grant from the Patient-Centered Outcomes Research Institute (PCORI) is enabling them to look at the decision-making journey by trying to obtain patient information before they need to make cancer screening decisions and seeing how that influences care. With a National Cancer Institute (NCI) grant, they are going to disseminate the MyPreventiveCare portal to 300 practices, many of them with low-literacy patients, in places such as inner city Richmond, Virginia, and among Native American and Hispanic populations in New Mexico.

So far, some 70,000 patients in 14 practices using 3 different EHRs have used MyPreventiveCare, and Krist noted that the number of patients is significant because it represents about 60 percent of patients in those practices. Between 50 and 100 new users sign up each week, he added. Krist said his team have had some trouble integrating into some commercial portals and that some practices are fielding two sites, their normal portal for emailing patients and disseminating lab results, and this one for preventive care. In those practices, about one-third of the patients use the normal portal, while two-thirds use MyPreventiveCare, reflecting the information needs of those patients. Across these practices, MyPreventiveCare accesses 22.9 million patient variables, and accounts for 176,742 unique EHR values and 4,941 prevention values.

In terms of what they have learned from the randomized controlled trial (Krist et al., 2014), the most important lesson has been that giving patients specific, tailored information helps them to act on preventive care. "They were more likely to go and get recommended care including screening and immunizations, and we saw increases of 12 to 16 percent for breast and colon cancer screening," said Krist. In some practices, breast cancer screening rates were already high, yet this type of information increased those rates to what may be a ceiling, which Krist called encouraging. Another finding was that not only is it important to get patients onboard, but getting clinicians onboard had a synergistic effect. "Half of the increase was probably from patient activation and the other half was from clinician activation," explained Krist. He added that patient summaries were sent to clinicians, leading practices to update 59 percent of patients' medical records and contact 84 percent of patients for further action, such as scheduling wellness or chronic care visits, or arranging for specific services.

This study also showed that patient need is substantial. In primary care settings, for example, users were up to date with only 53 percent of preventive care services. Only 2.2 percent of users were up to date on all services. On average, users who were not up to date needed 4.6 services, and in a separate study, using a health risk assessment plus tool, Krist and his collaborators found that patients on average had 5.8 unhealthy behaviors or mental health risks of the 13 items that they assessed. He noted that the practices that are using MyPreventiveCare today serve mostly higher-literacy populations, and despite being told by grant reviewers that this approach would only work with young healthy individuals who are technologically savvy, Krist and his team have found that a wide range of patients are willing to engage online. "Our highest user group was ages 55 to 65 and our second highest group was ages 65 to 75," said Krist. "Our lowest was the 20- to 40-year-old user group." Chronic disease, he said, appears to drive the highest level of use.

One of the challenges he and his colleagues encountered was getting information to patients at the right time, so the research team tried to engage people by sending them alerts before visits to have them review information and prepare themselves to be partners in making decisions about cancer screening, for example. This worked to some extent, but Krist said that further work is needed in the area of culture change to better integrate this process into the normal workflow. Another challenge has been to personalize content, and part of the PCORI-funded study involves asking patients who get breast, prostate, and colon cancer screening to think about and identify the information that they find most important. Focus groups with 100 patients identified the topics that were important, and fielding the content in MyPreventiveCare showed that most patients want that information in written form rather than as numbers, pictures, or stories. "I always hear that stories are great for conveying messages, but we're finding a lot of our patients want words," said Krist. "We're going to be looking at this and seeing what information people access and try to think of new ways of presenting this information." He concluded his comments by noting that there is some theory that suggests that if they do this right, this type of patient portal could reduce some health disparities, but that is something that remains to be tested and demonstrated.

REACTIONS TO THE PANEL PRESENTATIONS[4]

As a preface to his remarks, Dean Hovey explained that when he joined Digifit 4 years ago, the company's focus was on developing a device and app for heart rate monitoring that individuals could use to track their fitness and improve their performance. That, however, was not what Hovey wanted to do, so he changed the company's direction to one that developed health and wellness products that would help people learn health habits. His early background, he noted, was in product design and so he appreciated the importance of user experience. The dilemma he faced, though, is that making money in the mobile app arena is difficult because of the need to get millions of users to download the app for free and then convert some small subset of that population into customers who will pay for a premium service. "I actually wanted to get out of that business because it's really hard to make money giving away free apps."

The company began looking at human behavior and specifically at pregnancy because it represents a niche in which the users are young, technologically savvy, and social. Moreover, the users are hungry for information along a timeline that is predictable with the progress of their pregnancy. The challenge was to create an interactive design that will keep a user engaged for the 9 months of pregnancy to help her make good decisions. Pregnancy, as is the case with many chronic diseases, is something that tends to motivate people to take action and seek information.

The solution that Digifit created is a platform that enables them to create what they call an experienced design, which allows them to identify the target audience and the desired outcome and then develop a story arc that keeps them involved with the app. This process involves bringing together experts in the domain of interest with potential users, going into the homes of the audience that the app is intended to influence, and understanding the kind of information they need, what they need to pay attention to, and who the members of their social network are. They then put these pieces together to create a successful story arc. The Digifit platform also enables the developers to track what users are doing or not doing, which then allows them to engage in an iterative design process.

What he has learned from this process is that not only is it important to consider the needs of the individual, but of the care team involved with that individual. "You have to create social technical change with the care providers," said Hovey. "Most providers have never been in a place where they had 24/7 data and have been able to get into a person's home, so I

---

[4] This section is based on the comments of Dean Hovey, an experienced entrepreneur and currently president and chief executive officer of Digifit; Catina O'Leary, president and chief executive officer of Health Literacy Missouri; and Lana Moriarty, director of the ONC's Office of Consumer eHealth.

think that's the big piece here: How do you dive deep and interact and then make that information available?"

Catina O'Leary, who explained that she was representing the nonprofit sector, said her reaction to the three presentations was to wonder how her small company doing nonprofit work can engage at the intersection of companies and people. She noted that Health Literacy Missouri's offices are in a start-up incubator in St. Louis called T-Rex. When she tries to explain to the other companies working there what she and her colleagues do, they seem perplexed and cannot figure out how that fits and what a partnership would be like. "Figuring out what those relationships look like and how we can inform and participate is important," she said.

To some degree, it is great to hear people talk about going into homes and doing this work, said O'Leary, but her experience doing community-engaged research has been that the people who need the most help are reluctant to let researchers into their homes. "So how do we then also speak for the most vulnerable in our communities when that's appropriate, and what do those links look like? That's one of my most relevant reactions," O'Leary said.

Her other major comment, based on the work that her organization is doing, is that what people are really struggling with these days is figuring out the new health insurance laws and the benefits they are entitled to now that they have insurance. She told a story of a recent encounter she had with the health system, a first-time visit to the emergency room with her 6-year-old. She had called the phone nurse on a Sunday and was told based on her child's symptoms to go to the emergency room rather than urgent care. The result was a $300 bill, which O'Leary said was fine and understandable, but when she thought about people who do not have the resources that she has, it made her ask a number of questions. "How do people figure out what they need to know? How do they show up with the resources that they need? Where's the technology piece for that?" she asked.

She noted that one thing she and her colleagues have been hearing in Missouri is that people are using the periods outside of open enrollment to understand their health insurance and they are going back to the navigator who enrolled them to ask direct questions. The navigators often do not have answers and do not even have the information needed to answer those questions anymore. "I think we need to be talking about who these apps are for," said O'Leary, adding that while there is a need for consumer apps, there is also a need for apps for the providers, many of whom may not be trained in areas such as ethics and privacy.

The final reactor, Lana Moriarty, said that Holman's comment about looking to the private sector for innovations sums up the way ONC approaches much of its work in the field of health literacy. "We try to find the best practices, try to bring those to the table, make sure the right people are at the table," said Moriarty. She recounted her time working for the Health Resources and Services Administration (HRSA) in the field with underserved populations and remarked that it is important when thinking about digital health literacy to recognize that a significant proportion of the U.S. population struggles with computer literacy. She noted, too, that her team from ONC had a recent conversation with a provider in Tennessee who was meeting the meaningful use criteria, but whose major issue was that most of that practice's patients did not have computers and had no idea what computer to buy. In addition, while patients may have had smartphones, they may not have been downloading apps. "We need to consider that perspective," she said.

She commented how she was thrilled that the three speakers looked at how consumers and patients are really using technology, identifying the type of information they need, and then designing their apps and websites accordingly. "I appreciate the fact that this is about a user-centered experience and user-centered design," said Moriarty. "That is a key point." She reiterated the point that Holman made regarding the need to have intelligently structured data, without which there is the risk of having people misinterpret information and perhaps act on misinformation. "It is so hard to navigate across disparate sources of information," she said.

Moriarty said she was happy to see healthfinder.gov taken to a new level with MyPreventiveCare and was impressed with how many patients are using that portal. She said she wanted to explore with Krist issues of scalability and replicability, particularly because it appears that this portal breaks down some of the silos that have developed in the nation's health care system. "I know it wasn't the government's intention to create 10 different portals for your primary care physician and your different specialists, but that is the reality that we are living in now," she said. In fact, her team has been looking at an architecture that wraps data around a person instead of having it spread across disparate places, so she is eager to talk more about how to make that happen.

DISCUSSION

To start the discussion session, Suzanne Bakken asked the panelists and reactors if they had ideas on how to create a story arc for the use of consumer-facing technologies that takes health literacy into consideration, and if so, what some of the key targets for that story should be. O'Leary responded that the answer to this question relates to her comment that partnerships are important. "There's not one health literacy and there's not one story to tell," she said, which is why it is such a complex undertaking to communicate information across all kinds of conditions and accounting for all the different levels of understanding, from the patient to the physician and the health care organization. One challenge lies in the fact that many of those developing apps have never heard the term "health literacy" and have no idea of how to develop an app that has a foundation in health literacy. "So how do we make what we're doing become more central to the conversation, because it's not right now?" asked O'Leary. "We're still an emerging discipline, as much as we hate to admit that. So with that, are we really surprised that app creators don't know how to include this? Of course they don't."

That reality, in fact, is why Hovey's company has created a tool for app development given that app developers in general are not the subject matter experts. What needs to be done, said Hovey, is to give app developers the ability to merge their expertise with the experience of the health experts. As an example, he noted how an experienced heart surgeon has had conversations with hundreds of patients about what surgery and postsurgical recovery will entail. That surgeon understands that the conversation with each patient and the patient's family will be different based on what each patient hopes to gain from having surgery. This need to personify the message based on who the target is and what each individual's experience will be as far as what kind of information they get from an app does create a challenge. The surgeon may not have time to personalize that experience, but a nurse practitioner could help a patient download an app, provide instruction on how to use it, and set it up in a way that meets the needs of that specific patient.

Rosof asked how the health care team is going to find the time to educate patients about the use of technology, and Krist replied that there is, in fact, not enough time. The goal, though, is to integrate technology into the care setting so that it produces a net time savings. For example, his group has been trying to use the content that is coming from the patient experience to create standing orders for practices that will save time. In some cases, he said, these standing orders enable practices to use their secretarial and medical records staffs to call patients and offer them preventive services. "We've been trying to shift who is doing activities within practices as part of our strategy," said Krist, who added that he believes "there are many untapped opportunities where promoting health literacy, building teams, sharing information, and creating partnerships can really change what we can do."

Wendy Nickel, director of the ACP's Center for Patient Partnership in Healthcare, commented that 30 percent of ACP members are still in solo practice even with the move toward patient-centered medical homes and care teams. "These practitioners who are in solo practice don't have the time to sit down with their patient and go through their apps."

Hovey added that smartphones may not be the answer for all patients—the means to deliver this technology could be television and a remote control—and the key to success will be to deliver the technology and experience based on the needs of individual patients. Moriarty agreed with this last comment and with the idea that it is not likely to be the doctor who is teaching the patient how to download an app or use a particular technology tool. She added that her team has been studying how patients contribute to and manage their health care, what their goals are, and how they account for those life goals. If the whole point of being healthy is for a person to be able to do what he or she wants for as long as possible, asked Moriarty, at what point is it possible to create a story arc that enables an individual to use one of these technologies to help plan what to do to meet that goal and to become a partner with the entire care team?

Krist noted that patient stories are important for providing an understanding of the patient's perspective, and one of the things he has learned from his team's work is the importance of getting a breadth and depth of input. "In many of our studies, we have patients that we really partner with and they function with us as co-investigators and co-developers," said Krist. "We get really intensive input from them." He added that it has been important to see how these patients' stories change over time as they experience the health care system, and he also noted the importance of generating the evidence that a particular kind of input is beneficial. "The doctor in me quivers at 24 hours of patient data, and on the one hand I want it, but on the other hand, I want it only if I can act on it and it's going to improve things for my patients and make them better," he explained. In the same vein, the idea of having informaticians in his office mining these data is fine as long as the cost is balanced by how useful it is to have that kind of intense data analysis at hand. "I believe a lot of this is helpful, but I also believe it's our job to prove it's helpful before we advocate for it on big scales," said Krist.

Schnall commented on Holman's observation about how consumers rely on the Internet for their health information and noted that participants in her team's research have said they find answers to health-related questions from a doctor on Yahoo Answers. Part of the health literacy challenge, then, is to move past the idea that the prettier the website, the better the information must be. A shortage of information is not the problem, but helping people who can freely access information via their smartphones or computers to understand that information is a major challenge. To put that challenge in context, Holman said there are more than 40,000 Google searches per second, with 1 of every 20 of those searches health related, and while Google is the dominant player in the search field, it only accounts for about 58 percent of all searches.

Holman then remarked that he has a problem with the phrase "health literacy" because it implies to him that the problem is with the user. In his mind, the challenge is not to teach the public how to understand health messages, but to make health messages understandable from the start. As an example, he said that nobody talks about energy literacy, but the energy field has made a great deal of effort, led by the private sector, to educate people about their energy usage. Well-designed technology can help when it conveys useful information in such a way that users do not even realize they are engaging in a learning experience. In such cases, the usage experience is so intuitive that it becomes routine and natural enough to then have an impact on behavior.

Ruth Parker, professor of medicine, pediatrics, and public health at the Emory University School of Medicine, asked the panelists to describe what the public needs to understand today about privacy, data, and electronic health information. Hovey said it would be helpful if the people who wrote the explanations in the privacy notices of how data are going to be used did so in a simple format that says, "We're going to do this, this, and this, and we're not going to do this, this, and this," he said. The Apple research kits, he said, have done a good job of doing just that.

Social networking and crowdsourcing and how they enable patients and end users to share information can be powerful tools, said Schnall, but at the same time it is necessary to consider privacy and security. A challenge for the roundtable, she said, is to think about how to use those kinds of tools as a source of information and as a means of providing information through venues such as support groups for patients living with or at risk of disease while maintaining privacy and data security. Hovey cited pregnancy as an example of where the privacy issue is important and changing. During the first trimester, pregnancy is a secret, but as the pregnancy progresses the circle of who is in the know grows ever larger. "You have to be aware of that and you have to be aware of the spouse, the friend, the community advisor, the doctor, the nurse practitioner, and with each of those you need to have a unique view into the world of the patient," said Hovey.

Moriarty said she would be remiss if she did not mention the Blue Button connector website (bluebuttonconnector.healthit.gov), which was created as a one-stop shop for consumers to understand their legal rights to their electronic health information and to better prepare themselves for conversations on the topic with their health care team. The site was launched in September 2014 and already has 600 members who have committed to open data and giving consumers access to their data. It is also a place where consumers can find out about different apps that are on the market and how to aggregate and manage their health information. Bakken explained that there would be more time to discuss privacy and data access during one of the afternoon sessions of this workshop.

Michael Paasche-Orlow commented that intuitive design is in the eye of the beholder. He recounted a story of trying to get his 80-year-old father, who went to Harvard Law School and still practices law, to use his smartphone to take a picture of his mother, whose face was swollen after surgery.

"My head almost exploded in the process of trying to get him to do this," said Paasche-Orlow, "so intuitive design may be intuitive to you, but you actually have to find your target audience, understand what they can do, and figure it out."

Turning to the subject at hand, Paasche-Orlow said that although it is important to focus on knowledge and information exchange, people are not going to use an app unless it makes their life better, and so the main issue is function—what an app can do for an individual. "Can I make it so that I don't have to go to the pharmacy 10 times this month and instead synchronize all my medications to get picked up on the same day? That would make my life better," he said as an example of something a useful app could accomplish. Technology, he said, needs to reflect the fact that health care is a service industry, and that if all a technology does is transfer knowledge, it will not gain long-term use. Schnall added that it is not just a question of whether an app makes a person's life better, but if it is designed in a way that is entertaining, interesting, and compelling. She cited the fact that people waste hours playing games on their smartphones despite the fact that doing so does not make their lives better. "It's thinking about the functionality that our end users need that will help them continue using an app," she said.

For Krist, functionality is about making life easier. For example, an app that can better prepare a patient for a doctor's appointment and make the encounter a better use of time would be one that would make life easier. One thing that he has seen is that people get invitations to enter information into a portal to share with their doctor, but that they do not do so until after the visit, suggesting that perhaps the visit is a place where the physician can reinforce how much that information would have been useful to have beforehand. In that regard, he wondered if having thousands of apps in the market is a good thing because different approaches work for different people.

Rosof asked if the story arc can create cultural change by putting technology into play. Hovey said that can certainly help, but that smartphones and computers are not going to work with everyone. Today, he noted, a significant percentage of the population that most needs health information grew up in an era of radio and analog technology, and that group of people is likely to be more comfortable with a different type of user interface. One approach might be to change the reimbursement system to encourage health systems to deploy remote technology that would be useful to an elderly population instead of building new buildings. Until the health care enterprise starts thinking about software investments, which is about people and experiences, it will struggle with getting useful information to the population that needs that information the most today.

Terry Davis, professor of medicine and pediatrics at the Louisiana

State University Health Sciences Center, asked Hovey if he could teach the workshop something about what makes icons intuitive given that icons are important in health literacy. Hovey replied that it is important to remember that "you don't need an icon for everything," and he cited Apple's use of a button that says "next" instead of trying to come up with an icon that conveyed the same idea. "Sometimes we icon everything and it's not always easy to create an icon that communicates across the board," said Hovey. One of the features built into Digifit's system is that it records everything the user taps on their smartphone so that the developers can know if they used a particular feature and used it correctly. This capability, which is enabled by the Google App Engine and the company's ability to query large amounts of data, is showing that sometimes words work well and sometimes words plus an icon works better. He also noted that words may be needed only during the initial learning phase for an app.

Holman noted that jargon is often a middle layer between icon and plain language, and that there is often a period when a concept is introduced that requires simplicity. He explained that consumer brands deal with this problem regularly. He reminded the workshop that the Starbucks logo has undergone changes over time to reflect the fact that they needed to first introduce the lady on the logo and get people to associate that the lady equals Starbucks. "There's a mental translation between icon or brand and plain language, and I think where we the experts get stuck is in that middle layer, where we try to use words, but we're actually using jargon. It's a shortcut for us to mean something that through more words could actually be in plain language," said Holman.

Adriana Arcia, assistant professor at the Columbia University School of Nursing, said that she has been working with Bakken to develop infographics that can help a largely Dominican immigrant population with low health literacy understand patient-reported outcomes (Arcia et al., 2015). This has been an iterative process involving an interactive, participatory design exercise with the community, and the results have been surprising, she said. "We developed all kinds of different graphics using icons, and they were largely unsuccessful, especially anything that used repeated icons to represent multiple instances of any particular thing, such as servings of fruit," said Arcia. What did work, she said, is stars because games have taught people to rate things on a five-star system. "If the icons are really ubiquitous, if we've been trained to use them, then they're going to be successful."

Arcia then asked the panelists if they had any examples of assumptions that did not pan out. Holman replied that his office at one time ran competitions with cash prizes to spur the development of health-related apps. The competitions did accomplish that, but the surprising finding was that the developers were not taking the apps to market; they were just taking the cash prizes and going off and doing other things. "So it's a struggle in the world of open innovation to build sustainability into business models, and we're still trying to figure that out," said Holman.

Laurie Francis, senior director of clinical operations and quality at the Oregon Primary Care Association, reminded the workshop that the emphasis on training needs to be on the entire clinical team, not just the physician, and that the end user is actually the consumer, not the clinical team. She then asked about the relationship between the profit motive and the private sector and the fact that the people who most need this kind of help often do not have the money to pay for apps and the like. "Capitalism isn't looking for the consumer who has no money," she said, wondering how to create products for those who are most predisposed to poor health. Hovey responded with an example. Digifit is working with a group that provides in-home and clinic-based dialysis, and many of its clients are low-income individuals who cost the government some $60,000 per year just for dialysis. If Digifit can design an app that allows more of these individuals to receive less expensive in-home care and involve family members to provide part of the care, there may be an opportunity for the company to carve out some of the resulting savings.

Laurie Myers, lead for health care disparities and health literacy strategy at Merck, asked if the change in payment models that is occurring is creating opportunities to finance the need to put these technologies into the hands of those who need them most. Holman agreed that the shifting payment system is creating massive opportunities from a strictly capitalistic business perspective, particularly when juxtaposed with the incredible pace of technological change and the rate at which technology continues to become less expensive over time. He noted that Apple's deliberate decision to position itself at the high end of the market is a reflection of the fact that technology is going to get cheaper and that the market for these products will grow as a result.

Myers noted that she has been struck with the obligation of the field to think differently about the system and reduce complexity in a way that will enable disparate populations to take advantage of these technologies. Along those lines, she wondered if there are lessons from the gaming sector that might provide some insights into how to make these apps more universally attractive to end users. Hovey replied that one important lesson from the gaming industry is that many of the games are modular. "When they decide to add a new feature they snap it in and give it a 2- or 3-day test run, and if people use it, it stays in the game and if not, they remove it," he explained. Holman said that games are wholly immersive and that making information available through that sort of immersive experience is important.

Moriarty noted what an exciting time this is from her perspective given how many different factors are coming together, particularly with regard to the increasing number of consumers who are using portals to access their health information and the changing reimbursement structure that will increase data sharing across health care systems. "If we're going to get interoperability, we need more end users in the system and more people demanding for it to change," she said. Interoperability, she explained, is really about the ability to have data when and where the consumer needs it. The more consumers ask for their data and the more they demand that all the members of their health care team have access to their data, the more pressure will be brought to bear to make interoperability the norm.

Krist added that changing reimbursement policies are creating an opportunity for technology to help shift the cost curve as accountable care organizations take root and the demand for care coordinators, case managers, and patient navigators, many of whom have health literacy issues themselves, grows. Myers agreed and said that technology aimed at these new members of the health care team can help address these health literacy issues.

Nickel asked if the health care technology industry was going to help clinicians find the appropriate apps, out of the 40,000 or more available, that will support shared decision making between clinicians and their patients. Schnall noted that she and a colleague recently completed a review and analysis of existing mobile phone applications for health care–associated infection prevention (Schnall and Iribarren, 2015) and found there were 19 apps available. Of these, 18 provide only information, which she said is no different from picking up a book and reading the current guidelines on health care–associated infections. Only one of the apps provided feedback. She said that while she has not reviewed all 40,000 apps, she guessed that there is not a great deal of depth and richness in the health-related apps that are available. "We know that technology can be an enabler for helping people change their behaviors, but we're not developing technology that is an enabler for changing behaviors," said Schnall. This will only happen, she said, by going back to the drawing board and including end users and the entire care team in designing technology that can actually help people help themselves. Bakken noted that this topic would be discussed further in an afternoon session.

Wilma Alvarado-Little, principal and founder of Alvarado-Little Consulting, asked the panelists and reactors if they have any ideas about how to bridge the difference between someone being overwhelmed by the complexity of an app and noncompliance. Moriarty said she has been talking with health care providers who have told her there is a need to look at individuals who are given the opportunity to access their health data electronically, but do not take advantage of that opportunity. "Are we saying they're not interested? Are we saying there's no consumer demand for the information? Are we artificially suppressing demand by some of our workflow or by the cumbersome ways in which they may be accessing those data?" asked Moriarty. Answering those questions is important, she said, because it is the only way to fully understand what consumers want and how they can best access it according to their capabilities and needs, not those of the app developers.

Krist added that his group has some data showing that doctors may not think that their patients will use a technology at first, but then something happens, a few patients start using the portal or an app. Suddenly the doctor realizes that his or her patients will use the system and there is an avalanche of use. The challenge there is that patients ultimately get to decide whether they use technology or not. Doctors cannot be gatekeepers preventing use and if patients chose not to use technology then practices may suffer on some performance measures.

Erin Kent, program director in the Outcomes Research Branch of the Healthcare Delivery Research Program at NCI, noted that recent research (LeBlanc et al., 2014) found that having technology in the examination room can either improve a patient–provider encounter if the provider's baseline communication quality is already high, or it can actually hinder the social connection and communication that goes back and forth between the patient and provider if it is low. She also noted that studies of automated symptom reporting systems found that it is critical for patients to have access to a live human being on the other end of the phone and not just a recording. In that context, she asked if the panelists and reactors were thinking about how technology can be used to activate the human social component that patients need to change behavior. Holman responded that this is probably the right question to wrap up this discussion because one of the fundamental tenets of interacting with customers is talking to them, being able to have meaningful conversations, and being able to communicate in a way that works for them. "That's true whether you're talking about building an app or talking about teen pregnancy prevention," said Holman. He noted, though, that the technology space is not aiming at getting humans to interact with each other, but at understanding how to build the human components and the personification of human qualities into technology as a means of engendering trust that the information being delivered is useful and meaningful.

Moriarty commented that she has been seeing a growing number of hospitals and provider networks that are developing innovative ways of integrating social data into their EHRs with the goal of being able to show a patient in a limited amount of time that they care about them as a person. As examples, she cited the Chicago-based organizations that are making a database of community resources available to physicians so that they can put their clients who may have just lost a job or have to find a new place to live in touch with resources that can help them, and a physician in Washington, DC, who is connecting his low-income and migrant populations to parks near their homes so that they can get their families engaged in health-promoting activities. "Those are examples of how we're using technology to bring the human element into the exam room and the clinical setting," said Moriarty.

Hovey said his dream is to outfit a physician with a tablet that can provide distilled information on what the patient has done since last being seen to determine if the patient followed through on any recommended actions. Such an app would enable the physician to then focus on the items that still needed action. He then told a story about his recent encounter with a retinal surgeon, who he had gone to see because he had a retinal tear that needed repair. The surgeon sat down at his computer and had his back to Hovey, so Hovey decided to engage him and started asking him questions. The result was that the two of them engaged in a conversation on things that Hovey found important, but this episode illustrates the point that most doctors need training when they are also using a computer in the examination room, on how to engage their patients in a way that is most meaningful.

In closing the discussion, Rosof said that what he heard is that one of the most valuable attributes in the doctor–patient relationship or the health care team–patient relationship is trust. "So the question is, how can technology build trust? We have to think about that because we can't lose the trust piece, which is probably part of the time piece," said Rosof.

4

Catalyzing Widespread Informed Engagement

The workshop's second panel presented three aspects of how consumer-facing technologies can catalyze widespread informed engagement with the health care system. Patricia Dykes, senior nurse scientist and program director for research in the Center for Patient Safety Research and Practice and the Center for Nursing Excellence at Brigham and Women's Hospital and assistant professor at Harvard Medical School, discussed the skills that health professionals need to interface with consumers regarding consumer-generated information. Lygeia Ricciardi, principal of Clear Voice Consulting, then spoke about how digital health tools can create incentives for consumer engagement in health care. Alison Rein, senior director for Evidence Generation and Translation at AcademyHealth, addressed some of the ethical, legal, and social issues that are associated with consumer eHealth and big data. An open discussion moderated by Bernard Rosof followed the three presentations.

CONSUMER-GENERATED HEALTH INFORMATION: PROVIDER "READINESS," ATTITUDES, AND SKILLS[1]

Patient-generated health information, explained Patricia Dykes, is health information that is created, recorded, gathered, or inferred by or

---

[1] This section is based on the presentation by Patricia Dykes, senior nurse scientist and program director for research in the Center for Patient Safety Research and Practice and the Center for Nursing Excellence at Brigham and Women's Hospital and assistant professor at Harvard Medical School, and the statements are not endorsed or verified by the IOM.

from patients or their designees to help address a health concern (Derring, 2013). Patients can submit health history or treatment history information, or they might submit symptom logs so that their health care team members can assess how their patients are doing with self-management. At Partners HealthCare, patients routinely report outcome data related to cardiac surgery and orthopedic surgery. One of the fundamental characteristics of patient-generated health information, continued Dykes, is that it is captured by patients, recorded by patients, and shared by the patients if they decide to do so. Many patients, for example, collect biometric data and they may or may not share with their provider.

Patients believe that submitting these data is important because they can help keep the EHR up to date, and because they can provide a more complete picture of the patient's status than the data typically collected in the context of a visit. For example, patients who report their blood pressure readings over time are giving their providers a more complete picture than the snapshot readings taken in the office. Updated medication lists give providers a view of not just what they ordered, but what patients say they are actually taking. Patient-generated data can also provide the care team with access to the patient's problems, concerns, goals, and preferences, which can then improve the care plan concordance between patients and the care team, Dykes explained.

Given that research has shown that when providers pay attention to patient-generated information it improves engagement and activation (Hibbard and Lorig, 2012), what are the skills and attitudes needed to promote this kind of attention? One attitude, perhaps an overarching attitude, said Dykes, is the value proposition of patient-reported health information: that it can help solve problems and provide key benefits that improve care. "I think one of the challenges is communicating this to providers so that they are willing to interface with patient-reported health information," said Dykes. "We think the value proposition is that with the rise of smartphone and mobile devices, patient interest in health information has really exploded. Patient attention to health information when the provider is paying attention, too, actually improves engagement, activation, health, and wellness." In particular, Dykes noted the work of Judith Hibbard, who has shown that patients who are activated are more likely to undertake positive health behaviors, have lower costs, and have better outcomes than patients who are not (Hibbard and Greene, 2013; Hibbard et al., 2015).

In addition to the attitudes related to the value proposition, communication skills are essential for providers interfacing with patient-reported health information, something that Dykes noted was discussed in the workshop's previous session. "Now, more than ever, providers need to have expert communication skills, both face to face and when using technological tools," she said. "They need to know how to identify decision opportunities, recognize those opportunities, and take advantage of them. They need to then take the time to engage the patient using decision aids so that the patient can participate in the decision making and understand the information in the level of health literacy that is appropriate for them. This type of communication requires both a change in attitudes and training for many health care providers." Dykes added that communicating with surrogate decision makers is another important concept that many clinicians need to learn. It comes into play when surrogates need to report patient information that the patients themselves are unable to report because of their medical condition or because of language barriers. At Brigham and Women's Hospital, for example, physicians and nurses engage care partners who are communicating for patients who are in intensive care and oncology units.

Assessment skills are also important when it comes to determining how health literate a particular patient may be, and the outcomes of these on-the-spot assessments should determine the types of tools that the care team uses with a particular patient. Again referring to research by Hibbard, Dykes noted that disease management improves when matching a patient's activation level with the care plan and using the activation level to determine the types of tools and the intensity of follow-up that is required for a patient (Hibbard et al., 2009).

Another important skill that the health care team requires is the ability to sort through patient-generated data. "There is a lot of fear about this," said Dykes. "Today, relatively few patients are contributing health information to their electronic record and submitting it to their providers. We need to adopt our informatics strategy so that we can process big data, not only taking these data in, but having the ability to display them in a way that they are going to be usable for clinical decision making." Currently, she explained, there is an active debate about whether or not data entered into the EHR require review. She noted that in preparing for this presentation, she spoke to many providers who told her that they do not want to see Fitbit data because they have no idea how they will process that information within the time constraints of the 15-minute office visit.

What the field needs, said Dykes, is a taxonomy to differentiate those data that need to be reviewed versus those data that patients can just submit into the EHR. To deal with those data that the patients do submit, the field needs to develop a workflow to make use of those data. In the Brigham and Women's Promoting Respect and Ongoing Safety through Patient-centeredness, Engagement, Communication, and Technology (PROSPECT) project, for example, Dykes and her colleagues thought carefully about the workflow needed to accommodate data from every piece of technology they implemented to ensure that any data a patient submitted would be considered by the health care team.

The PROSPECT project is one approach to addressing the provider skill set that is needed for processing patient-reported information in an acute care setting, in this case for patients receiving a bone marrow transplant or in the intensive care unit. PROSPECT is a cluster-randomized controlled trial that began in June 2014 and was scheduled to run through May 2015. Its goal is to optimize the overall experience of patients and care partners by facilitating engagement, improving care plan concordance, promoting dignity and respect, and enhancing satisfaction. The first of two important components to the intervention is the Patient SatisfActive Model, a structured team communication model that tries to improve patient experience and satisfaction in real time by giving providers the skills, tools, and workflow to improve communication between clinicians and patients and their family members. This training aims to promote attentiveness to the patient's needs, concerns, and expectations in real time, and to engage the patient and family in the decision making, paying attention to cultural diversity; and then looking closely at each patient's health literacy levels and how that determines the tools that the care team will use with a given patient.

The second component is a patient-centered, Web-based toolkit and microblog, essentially a Web portal where patients can report their overall goal for hospitalization, state their daily goals, and rate how well they think the care team is doing with their care (see Figure 4-1). Patients can also view the care team's goals, see problems that care team members have identified, and then provide feedback to the care team. Patients can also message their care team about their care plans at any time. PROSPECT also has a set of provider-facing tools that are designed to integrate the review of patient-reported information into the workflow. For example, the safety checklist component of this toolkit puts as its first item the ability of the nurse to present any new patient or family input from the Patient SatisfActive webpage or microblog. The provider-facing tools also serve as the interdisciplinary care plan platform where the care team reviews what the patient or family reports over the past 24 hours and then agrees on a strategy for addressing any concerns. "For example they discuss whether they are going to go in during rounds and talk to that patient and family, in a family meeting, or whether they are going to use the microblog and respond that way" Dykes asked.

Implementing the Patient SatisfActive Model has been successful and appears to be a reasonable approach, Dykes said, but there have been some challenges that PROSPECT had to address. Working with incapacitated patients and elderly, for example, requires engaging care partners to input information into the patient-facing Web portal. Workflow integration has gone well with teams based within the hospital, but has been less successful with non-local providers and consultants. PROSPECT has improved the ability to manage a multidisciplinary care plan by incorporating patient preferences, goals, and priorities and by reconciling siloed nurse and phy-

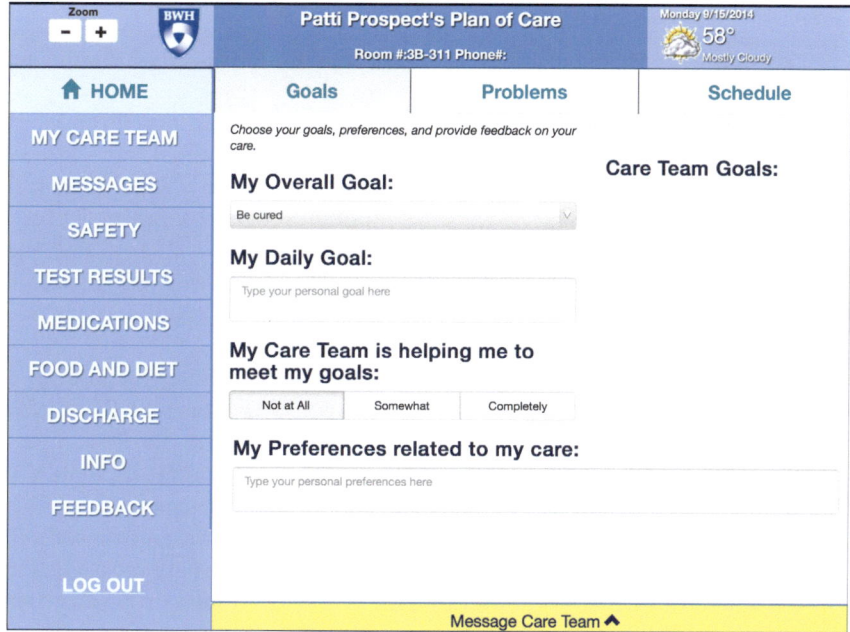

FIGURE 4-1 A patient-facing webpage from PROSPECT.
SOURCE: Dykes presentation, March 24, 2015.

sician documentation, but there is still room for improvement, she said. A major barrier when the project went live, and one that Dykes and her colleagues are still addressing, has been getting providers to understand the value of patient-generated information.

In conclusion, said Dykes, patient-generated health information can be used to inform care decisions and to promote shared decision making. "It is important that we first recognize the value of patient-reported health information and that we consider what the impact is going to be on workflow and address that as part of the project," she said. "Attention to provider readiness and logistical skills are key to success, and implementation is not without real-world challenges. True stakeholder engagement in designing the data, information, and workflows was an important preparatory activity that has helped us quite a bit through this project and continues to help us."

INCENTIVES FOR CONSUMER ENGAGEMENT[2]

Ricciardi discussed the consumer or patient perspective on the use of digital health tools. She started by discussing the tools available for increasing consumer engagement in their health care and noted that there is a rapidly growing number of consumer health apps, mostly monitoring exercise and diet, with some tied to wearable sensors or biometric devices. Forecasts project there will be some 68 million users of wearable electronic fitness monitoring devices worldwide in 2015 (Gartner, 2014), and that more than 70 million personal health and wellness devices will be sold in the United States alone by 2018, generating more than $8 billion in product sales and service revenues.

People are beginning to use these apps and wearables, according to research from the Pew Research Center (Fox and Duggan, 2013), but the potential for growth remains substantial. According to the Pew report, 69 percent of adults track their health or the health of others in some way (whether digitally or in a non-digital format), with the majority recording weight, diet, or exercise, but only 21 percent of trackers are using technology to track health. People with chronic health conditions are most likely to be trackers. Another study found that 10 percent of adults own an activity tracker, but that 50 percent who have owned one stop using it and 30 percent stop within the first 6 months (Ledger and McCaffrey, 2014). Ricciardi counted herself among those who own activity trackers that now sit unused in a drawer, though she added the devices still impacted her being engaged in her health. As an example, she said that after she had her first child, she joined an online weight-reduction program for only a few months, but from which she took lessons she is still using today. "I do not think that a measure of success for an app or a tool has to necessarily be that I have it strapped to my body forever," said Ricciardi.

The take-away from these figures is that people are using these technologies, but that they have not yet met their full potential. One question that needs addressing is how to learn more about what technologies people do or do not adopt. "How do we choose?" she asked. "Right now, there is no real guidance on what to use, and I would suggest that a potential role for the IOM might be to create a rubric or a framework through which public- and private-sector entities could come together and help develop a code for what is desirable in these technologies." In her opinion, the key characteristics of technologies are that they are useful, user-friendly, either good looking or invisible, comfortable, hardy, and affordable. They would also come with transparent privacy practices, integrate easily with other

---

[2] This section is based on the presentation by Lygeia Ricciardi, principal of Clear Voice Consulting, and the statements are not endorsed or verified by the IOM.

products, and be of a trusted brand with good reviews. She noted that one app she recently tried sent a text message to one of her friends telling her that this app was now mapping her runs. As far as she knew, the app never asked permission to do this and she would not have known it was doing so if her friend had not alerted her to the fact. "I was unhappy and I still hold it against that product," said Ricciardi. "I imagine that I'm not the only consumer who is going to feel incensed when we find our information is being used in ways that we were not informed about."

Besides her personal and informal list of desirable characteristics for an adoptable technology, there are other motivators for people to adopt apps, tools, and technologies, such as the fun factor and the extent to which the technology can be tailored to the user's personal health goals and preferences. Technologies that contribute to society, perhaps by enabling the user to contribute data to a pooled database for research or other purposes, are more likely to be adopted, too. As an example, she cited the fact that 80 percent of the clients of the genomics company 23andMe say they are willing to share their data for research.

There are also a number of extrinsic motivators that can encourage people to adopt or use some of these tools. Money is a big one, and potential sources include employers, payers, providers, and accountable care organizations. As an example, Ricciardi described the Welltok Health Platform, an app that employers can offer that gives people incentives such as coupons based on adoption of healthy behaviors. Castlight is an app that employers can provide to their employees to enable them to compare the cost of potential service providers, thus enabling them to realize financial savings. Other extrinsic motivators are social in nature, such as the app Stickk, which enables users to bet with their friends that they will meet some health-related goal, such as going to the gym a certain number of times per week. If the user does not meet the goal, the app donates money to a cause the user designates as one that he or she does not like.

With regard to what is on the horizon, Ricciardi believes there will be increasing use of extrinsic incentives. "I think we will see more of the major players, from providers to payers to affordable care organizations, who are motivated through policy changes to get consumers to be more engaged in their health," she said. She noted that she would like to see more evidence about what kinds of apps and tools are effective because that will help consumers choose among the thousands of choices, and she predicted that this evidence base will contribute to a market consolidation. Because health is so integrated into the rest of life, she predicted that the lines between health apps and tools and generic ones would blur. "You wouldn't think of having a separate designated health phone and a finance phone," she said, and she expected that more generic information, such as what a person buys at the grocery store, who is in their social network, and how often they interact with members of that network, might become part of a person's health information. In short, she said in conclusion, she was hopeful there will be "increased adoption and use of these tools in a way that they really become a ubiquitous part of our lives in a way that helps us reach the health goals we define as individuals."

BUILDING A FABRIC OF TRUST: ETHICAL, LEGAL, AND SOCIAL ISSUES IN THE ERA OF eHEALTH AND BIG DATA[3]

Alison Rein started the final presentation in this session by explaining that she oversees a portfolio of work at AcademyHealth that straddles two major focus areas. The first is how to use these new data sources, coming from both within and outside of the health care system, to generate better evidence. The second is how to engage patients and consumers more meaningfully in that evidence-generation process. She also emphasized just how important the ethical, legal, and social dimensions of "this brave new world of consumer eHealth" are to getting the most out of these new data sources.

To help provide some background to her talk, Rein explained that AcademyHealth envisions a future where individuals and communities are made healthy by the use of evidence in decision making. To realize this vision, the organization's mission is that, together with its members, it will work to improve the health and performance of the health system by supporting the production and use of evidence to inform policy and practice. The Electronic Data Methods Forum is one program that AcademyHealth believes will help it fulfill this mission. Funds for this project are part of a major infrastructure investment by the Agency for Healthcare Research and Quality (AHRQ) through the Health Information Technology for Economic and Clinical Health (HITECH) Act, enacted as part of the American Recovery and Reinvestment Act of 2009. The forum recognizes that with the increased use of EHRs, there is a potential gold mine of data and information in these systems. However, there are some thorny issues related to methods, governance, data quality, informatics, and the application to a learning health care system that must be addressed to tap the riches of this gold mine. The forum, which also recognizes that tackling each of these issues independently in their separate silos will take far too long to create a learning health care system, has created a learning community around these issues that engages people who are trying to use electronic health data for operational, quality improvement, and research purposes. "We use this as

---

[3] This section is based on the presentation by Alison Rein, senior director for evidence generation and translation at AcademyHealth, and the statements are not endorsed or verified by the IOM.

an opportunity to do collaborative work, to share insights, and to work on shared challenges together," said Rein.

Another initiative that AcademyHealth started some 4 years ago is called the Consumer Patient Researcher Roundtable, which again focuses on collaboration. "We recognized early that very often when we went to meetings, the interests of academics and researchers were presented as polar opposites from the views and interests of patients and consumers, which is actually odd when you think about it because I never met a researcher who said that he or she was trying to do things to the disadvantage of the patients he or she serves," said Rein. As a result, the roundtable promotes conversations and looks for opportunities in the eHealth space where researchers and consumers can work together.

Rein noted, as did Ricciardi, that while there has been a great deal of focus on the robust data streams coming from EHRs, there is an explosion of data from other sources, including devices, apps, and websites. "I think this is a golden opportunity for people where I sit, for the research community, and for pretty much everybody who cares about health because we can now look at data that go beyond the 10 percent of health that is represented by or attributable to what happens in the care experience and look at the 90 percent of health that is affected by everything else," said Rein.

The ability to use technology to better engage patients offers tremendous opportunities and potential benefits, said Rein, who noted several examples:

- Improved patient access to their own clinical information via providers and insurers.
- Engagement with health and wellness information via portals and websites.
- Enhanced quality and coordination of care.
- Expanded opportunity to contribute to and participate in research.
- Increased ability to "quantify self" via apps, wearables, and devices.

As Ricciardi and others mentioned, Rein said there is a tremendous appetite on the part of patients and consumers to engage in this space. A report from the PricewaterhouseCoopers Health Research Institute stated that 47 percent of consumers agree that mobile devices can be used more effectively to coordinate care, and that 65 percent of consumers with one or more health apps on their mobile devices use them at least once weekly. Half of the consumers surveyed said they would be likely to use consumer devices to perform self-evaluations and 56 percent said they would be comfortable having their health data shared if doing so would improve care coordination (PricewaterhouseCoopers, 2014). Rein noted that the ONC and the National Partnership for Women and Families each released survey results over the past year that corroborate and extend these findings.

Given the appetite consumers have for eHealth applications, it is important to consider the risks and whether those risks are evenly distributed across all constituents. Loss of privacy is the risk that gets the most attention and it can take two forms: (1) personal identification and blind discrimination, or (2) discrimination by association. As an example of the former, Rein noted how purchasing an item online suddenly seems to trigger a host of related content appearing on other websites. Discrimination by association refers to a characteristic that a person might have that is associated with something else, such as prior incarceration. Another risk is loss of control of one's own information, and to some extent, this may have happened already. Diminished access to potentially beneficial information or treatment is a risk that is associated with the fact that many vulnerable populations may not get access to care because they cannot purchase an app or device and have to relinquish some level of control in order to gain access to something they believe they need medically. Rein said these risks are not evenly distributed.

There is no comprehensive framework for health information privacy and security, Rein said. Although this has been said many times, it bears repeating, she explained. Societal norms informed by the Hippocratic Oath, together with legal protections afforded by the Health Insurance Portability and Accountability Act (HIPAA), the Genetic Information Nondiscrimination Act (GINA), and the Common Rule, are only in force for data generated by the health system. For patient- and consumer-generated data, there are few protections and many points of potential risk, a situation that Rein characterized as being like the Wild West.

"Given all of this," said Rein, "I think the question becomes what things are health literacy sensitive? That is, if we apply basic health literacy concepts and practices, could we reasonably expect consumers to take some different action? Conversely, are there things that are so complex or so opaque or where there is no transparency that it is just really too much to expect that consumers would be able to engage or interact in that way?" Consumer use of mobile apps provides one example of something that is potentially health literacy sensitive. Mobile apps, websites, and devices all capture the users' data, and in many cases are contributing data to a larger, aggregate dataset from others who happen to use those technologies. In large part, explained Rein, these data are aggregated, de-identified, and then used for a variety of purposes. "There is some commoditization happening on the back end that is important to recognize."

Consumers, said Rein, need to look for "terms of use" and privacy statements for each app they use; they need to determine if their own data are accessible; and they need to assess the sensitivity of the data being shared. Designers, on the other hand, need to make "terms of use" and privacy statements easily accessible and understandable, and they need to share back and contextualize data to users. "There are some vocal ePatient advocates who are frustrated by the fact that they cannot extract their own data from some of these devices," said Rein. Designers should also solicit user feedback in the design process, particularly from users with lower health literacy, and build in feedback design loops to the process.

Consumer participation in research or voluntarily donating data for research is another health literacy–sensitive area that holds a great deal of promise for generating advances, particularly in light of the release of Apple's research kits. In addition to looking for "terms of use" and privacy statements and determining if their own data are accessible, consumers need to assess the value of participation in a given research project. Designers need to follow the same guidelines that they do for apps, plus they need to improve processes, pathways, and the use of informed consent. Rein noted that some entities doing research are covered by HIPAA regulations, but some are not, and she said following HIPAA would be a good health literacy design standard for the field to adopt.

She also noted that many of the vehicles used today for informed consent do not really do the matter justice. She mentioned a project that the Electronic Data Methods Forum conducted with John Wilbanks at Sage Bionetworks to create a set of wire frames and extractable components that can be used to obtain consent via a mobile device. Some of these components were included in Apple's research kit. This participant-centered consent toolkit uses icons and words to walk the participant step by step through the consent process and test the user's understanding of consent at each step.[4]

A less clear area of concern entails consumers searching for information on health-related websites. More than 70 percent of American adults look up health information online, but only 36 percent know that advertisers are allowed to track their visits to health-related websites. Moreover, some 77 percent of searches begin not at a health-related website such as WebMD, the National Institutes of Health (NIH), The Mayo Clinic, or AHRQ, but at Google, Bing, or Yahoo. Most of these searches track back to large corporations, such as Google and Facebook, and to data brokers, such as Experian and Acxiom. These are what is known as third party requests. First party requests, explained Rein, are those in which the user gets information directly from the website being visited, whereas third party requests are those for which the host website has to get information that it extracts from other sites. Those requests "leak" information on the user to the third parties, triggering privacy concerns.

---

[4] See http://sagebase.org/e-consent (accessed March 24, 2015).

"Is there a health literacy–sensitive solution to these concerns?" asked Rein. Her answer was "maybe." Her pessimism stems from the difficulty that the average person, including herself, would have in protecting his or her own data without help and the fact that add-on software solutions are themselves burdensome to end users. Even when done well, data protection is only moderately effective, claimed Rein. "Again, going out on a limb and being a bit provocative, this may be an opportunity where regulatory and/or policy solutions are needed."

DISCUSSION

Bernard Rosof started the discussion by asking panelists to comment on the key challenges they see in getting consumers to sustain their use of consumer-facing technology and on getting providers to use the data generated by their patients' use of the technology. Rein said that one general rule regarding consumer sustainability is that the technology needs to be easy to use without changing the consumer's workflow. If a device runs out of batteries, needs recharging constantly, or is hard to set up, the consumer is much more likely to drop it. She also thought that just as physicians do not want all of the data that a Fitbit generates, neither do consumers. "What we need is smart software that helps us interpret key changes in the data or that alerts us to pay attention to things because we are going to be increasingly measuring and recording more data about every aspect of our lives, and none of us is going to want to review it all," said Rein. "What are some ways that we can use intelligent technology to make sense of the data and highlight useful key points? That will be worthwhile."

A workshop participant agreed with those points and added that there needs to be a return on investment for both the patient and the provider; one way to increase the return on investment would be with the kind of software that Rein described. Such software, said the participant, needs to support decision making, depending on who is using the data. Return on investment increases as the data become more usable and useful, and there is evidence, said the participant, that patients become activated and engaged in their health care when the data they provide are useful to their providers. "I do not think all providers know that and I do not think all providers understand exactly what patient activation is," said the participant. "These are all skill sets that I think we have to reinforce and teach." Rein then added that PatientsLikeMe reinforces the idea that patients give something and they get something back. "That has certainly helped keep a steady stream of people engaged in that site," she said.

Rein also noted that providers have a high threshold for evidence. "I have talked to many who say 'I want to know before I totally redesign my systems and my processes that I am going to get value from doing this,'" she explained. She also noted that the process of showing that particular types of patient-generated data are useful is going to be long and fraught with failure. The field needs to understand that some data will be useful, and some will be useless. Ricciardi added that there is an assumption that the categories or types of patient-generated health data will need to be approved before they goes into the EHR, but she and her colleagues do not think this is necessarily the case. "If patients want to report their goals or particular data sets that they believe contributed to meeting those goals, they should be free to do so. Discussing the goals and the data with health care providers will help patients and providers to better understand one another," said Ricciardi.

Bringing up the concept of behavioral economics and the way in which incentives were used with meaningful use, Rosof asked if a similar approach was going to be taken to encourage uptake of consumer-facing technology. Ricciardi predicted there will not be a meaningful use program for consumer health information technology. What she hopes will happen is that payment reform, particularly with regard to changing the underlying financial incentives in the health care system, will align the patient and provider in terms of having the goal of doing whatever is necessary to keep the patient healthy in an efficient way. "That, I think, will necessitate the engagement of consumers and individuals in their own health, which means relying on technology," said Ricciardi. "We rely on digital tools and digital information in every other industry and it just makes sense. More information enables us to make better decisions." She recounted that when she worked at ONC she found that not all stakeholders were afraid of patient-generated data. Many physicians, she said, wanted nothing to do with these data because they were not sure how to process it or how to be reimbursed for their time in doing so, while some of the major retail pharmacy chains were eager to have access to patient data and to use it to build stronger relationships with consumers.

Rosof then asked Rein to comment on how EHR data will be used. Her response was that they are being used today for quality improvement initiatives, comparative effectiveness research, and population health management. "A lot of characterizing of populations, of segmenting them, of trying to assign some type of risk, and of developing a proactive plan for mitigating risk is happening," she said. In the past, the need to wade through thousands of paper records to find the necessary information for such studies made them unreasonable to conduct. Rosof noted that "patients are actually contributing to society without really knowing about it," to which Rein said, "Sometimes, yes, unless they fully understand the HIPAA waiver." She suggested that for health literacy reasons, it might be a good idea to change that waiver so that it is more understandable to more people. Ricciardi added that while many people—both providers and patients alike—think that HIPAA prevents individuals from getting access to their own health data, the fact is that HIPAA guarantees everyone's right to access their own health information. That component of HIPAA, she said, should be just as well known as the privacy piece of HIPAA, but unfortunately it is widely misunderstood.

Ruth Parker added that she wanted to make one thing clear about how EHRs are being used: "Billings are improving and that is a big issue for patients. The EHRs that we have and that we use came to be because we addressed that part of it. I think we are in the embryonic phases of figuring out how they can be good and useful." Rosof asked Parker if EHRs could identify gaps in care that could lead to performance improvement and better outcomes. Parker replied that she believes this is possible and is being done is some places. She also stressed that while many institutions have built out their EHRs for the principles related to outcome and performance improvement, it is important to understand that the original interfaces were designed primarily for billings. Rosof remarked that there are four drivers of provider behavior: professionalism, performance, payment, and patients. "How you prioritize those seems to set institutions apart, and I think EHRs need to get up to that task."

Rosof asked the panelists to comment on the Apple research kit and how it might affect research. Will it skew the data? Will it lead to increased health disparities? What are the ethical and privacy implications of such a system? Rein replied that Apple has established a baseline level of setting expectations in terms of disclosures and privacy concerns for those who want to use the research kit. She also said that the question of skewing is an important one, but noted that she had heard some 48,000 people had signed up to participate in research projects in just the first few days the research kit was available. This suggests that this system might broaden participation. What could be skewed, she said, is that this system excludes users of the Android operating system, which happens to serve many potentially vulnerable populations. "There is now this pressure to build a comparable mechanism to conduct research and apply the same tools and framework to the Android space. I do not think it is going to be exclusively an Apple endeavor for long, at least based on the conversations that I am hearing," said Rein. "Then there are endless opportunities for far larger sample sizes than we have enjoyed in prior research efforts. Obviously, that means there is another set of methodological and other issues that are going to be triggered."

Ricciardi commented that Apple, because of its cache among consumers, is helping to put health on the map for the average person even though the average Apple user tends to have a higher income because the products are more expensive. "But I think their entrance into this space, combined with their skills at marketing and mainstreaming things, is changing mindsets so that people will associate health with their phone or watch and start feeling like these devices and apps and tools are part of the mainstream experience of their lives." Although traditional research will certainly continue, the opportunity is growing to augment traditional research with real-time data from people in their natural environments.

Rima Rudd, senior lecturer on health literacy, education, and policy at the Harvard School of Public Health, noted that there was a roundtable forum 5 or 6 years ago at which there was a discussion on ownership and control of data, particularly with regard to traveling population groups such as the homeless who might need to make a decision on what data they want to share with a clinician. That control and ownership were absent from this workshop's discussions so far, she said. Dykes said the question of ownership comes up frequently in the comments that patients submit to their microblog. Currently, in the research context, patients are not getting their data. She and her colleagues are exploring the recommendations and infrastructure needed to be able to provide patients with access to these kinds of data.

Ricciardi said she likes the model in which patients collect their health data and choose to whom to give access and how it will be used. "I tend to dislike the term 'ownership' in this particular context," she said. "I do not think anyone really owns data in an electronic environment in which it can be easily copied and dispersed." Instead, she prefers the idea of control, of giving the patient more control over how information is used rather than "going down the rabbit hole of discussing who owns something. It's a small shift in how we talk about it, but I would stay away from the term 'ownership' per se." Rein said the issue of who is allowed to do what, why, when, and in what context remains an overarching theme in much of the work she does. Health systems, she said, act as stewards of the data because they have a legal record that they are responsible for maintaining and they do maintain a higher standard for access and sharing through the Institutional Review Board mechanism. Outside of the health system, though, there are far fewer controls and probably less knowledge about controlling access to data. What Rein would like to see is that all data are returned to the individual and that some tool, which has yet to be developed, nicely organizes an individual's data and enables that person to authorize who gets access to those data.

Rudd then commented that health literacy is a two-sided coin. On one side is an individual's listening and comprehension skills, while on the other side is the health care provider's speaking and explanatory skills. "One cannot measure someone's listening skills without measuring the speaking skills, and one cannot measure literacy skills without understanding the difficulty and complexity of the various texts," she explained. In that context, she asked Dykes if her project includes an evaluation of both patient literacy skills and some measure that can differentiate if one team has better communication skills than another. Dykes replied that the research team did create a standard for communication and that providers are documenting when they address patient's needs, concerns, and expectations. What her team does, then, is track the frequency with which they document those factors during different phases of care, such as when they first enter the intensive care unit, when they are being treated, and when they are transitioning out of the unit. She noted that getting providers onboard with this requirement was a paradigm shift of sorts because the clinicians did not think this kind of information was valuable.

Parker asked the panelists if anyone has asked patients and consumers what they really care about with regard to privacy and data access. Rein said the only thing she knows is how much she does not know about what consumers want because it is wrong to assume that all consumers want the same thing. "I think there is a tendency to say patients and consumers all need and want the same thing, and my observation is just that there is a continuum. Depending on where you are in the continuum of your life and your health, your needs and expectations are going to be profoundly different," said Rein. "We need to be able to acknowledge that and design for that at the care level, the research level, and every level." She also acknowledged that this is not a satisfying answer to the question, but that it is the best that she has been able to come up with over the past 10 years.

Ricciardi said she agreed with Rein's assessment, but added that there are some generalizations to be made based on surveys of what people expect with regard to health care. For most people, their primary concern is to be well, and many do not want to think about their health or health care, especially if there is not a problem. Many individuals with a chronic condition do not want to identify as someone with a chronic condition. People also express real interest in having a greater connection to their physician and they want to communicate more. "They want to establish a closer relationship, rather than one based on a 15-minute visit once a year," said Ricciardi. Another obvious want is for health care to be easier, something that she identifies with as a mother of two children. "I hate that I have to drive in a rain storm, park my car, and bring my kid into the pediatrician just to show that she has that same eye infection that I knew she had because we've treated it in the past. If I could have just taken a picture with my smartphone, and if my doctor would trust me and would be reimbursed for prescribing whatever I needed to deal with the fact that she has pinkeye, everyone would be so much better off," said Ricciardi. "Make this much less difficult for us please!"

Earnestine Willis, the Kellner Professor in Pediatrics and director of the Center for the Advancement of Underserved Children and of Health Equity and Urban Clinical Care Partnerships at the Medical College of

Wisconsin, asked Dykes if the PROSPECT project was changing both what physicians were doing and how the institution was getting information into the community. Dykes replied that PROSPECT and other efforts are changing how the institution communicates with patients by providing the community with the tools that allow them to communicate with and purposefully engage care partners. She noted, too, that it is important to engage people in the community because their capacity to engage and be activated is much less when they are in the hospital. Moreover, unless the community is engaged, and that includes a patient's family and other potential caregivers, they are not going to be activated when they leave the hospital and return to the home and community setting. "In this project, we are trying not just to enroll the patient, but also to ask the patient who else can work with you to make sure that when you are not feeling well that we can still further your care plan and make sure that your goals are achieved," explained Dykes. She added that this is an attitude shift that she hopes is being communicated to the community, that Brigham and Women's Hospital is taking the time to not only engage the patient, but to make sure that others in the community are working with patients when they go home to further their care plan.

Willis also asked if the panelists have given any thought in this world of technology about issues of liability, given the recent data thefts that had occurred at two large health systems. Rein said this is certainly a concern and one that may be contributing to the reluctance of providers to absorb patient-generated data. She noted that Kaiser has been looking at what happens to patient-generated data once they have been integrated into the workflow and accepted into the EHR, but that this is an area that needs further exploration.

Suzanne Bakken asked the panel to speak about the idea of preparing the public, starting in kindergarten and running through high school, to participate in research studies using consumer-facing technologies. "Thinking about what we have been discussing today, what are the implications for clinician education in particular so that they can be integrating these tools into their practice more effectively?" she asked. Ricciardi strongly supported the idea of starting in the K-12 environment to create the mindset that everyone is welcome to participate in research and must be responsible for being more engaged in their health, and technology provides a set of tools to do that. She noted that when she was at ONC, there was a great deal of discussion about a shift in mindset being one of the biggest challenges facing the health care field. "What is required is not only changes in technology or payment reform—those are important pieces, too—but a shift in attitudes is really a critical piece of what we are talking about, and you really cannot start too early with that," said Ricciardi. She noted that ONC is conducting a big public relations campaign related to the Blue

Button initiative in partnership with a number of nonprofit organizations to get the word out and get people in the mindset that they need to be involved in maintaining and managing their own health. "But I would love to start talking about the individual's role relative to personal health earlier in schools as well," she said.

Dykes agreed that attitude change is important and that changing provider attitudes was an important early piece of her work. When she and her colleagues first started implementing the patient-centered toolkit, providers expressed concern that patients were going to be communicating with them. "They did not see the value of giving patients this much information, that it would make the patient anxious," said Dykes. It was necessary, she said, to make the case that engaging with patients was best done by providing them with the same information that the clinicians had, but in a way that would be useful to the patients, using resources such as Medline Plus. She also stressed the importance of obtaining provider input on workflow. "They have to be part of this. You have to hear their concerns and move with them," said Dykes.

Winston Wong noted that the Roundtable on the Promotion of Health Equity and the Elimination of Health Disparities was going to be holding a workshop that would discuss how to increase minority participation in clinical trials. He wondered if the panelists had given any thought about how health information technology could be used to facilitate the involvement of underserved populations in clinical trials. Ricciardi responded that ONC held a roundtable on this topic when she was working there. "One big take-away for me was that you need to involve a lot of trusted community organizations or other representatives of the communities that you are trying to reach. It could be a house of worship, a health care organization, or a school, anything that the folks you are looking to as a group consider a home or resource that they trust. They say health care is local, and it does revolve around particular cultural communities as well as geographic ones. Members of a given community will help you figure out how specifically to employ technology—it is going to vary based on what group you are talking with and their particular norms and expectations," said Ricciardi.

In a PCORI-funded project aimed at preventing falls, Dykes and her colleagues are running a clinical trial at 10 sites across the United States that involves a health information technology intervention. Nurses serve as fall care managers and make sure that patients receive and understand their assessments and tailored plans. The details for this intervention were worked out with the help of stakeholder councils that represented the different areas in which this research would be conducted. In some regions, particularly the Southwest, minorities are the majority and they formed these councils. "It is making sure that you are touching base with all the stakeholders that are going to be representing users of the technology and participants in the trial and addressing their concerns," explained Dykes. "We did that in preparation for submitting the application, but every month at every clinical trial site we continue to meet with these stakeholders and do refinements when we run into trouble."

Michael Paasche-Orlow said he helped to build an interactive voice response system that called parents before they brought their children in for an appointment. He asked the physicians how often they wanted to see the data that the parents provided to the system. The answer was never, he said. Nonetheless, the investigators automatically input the data into the clinic note and the physicians were thrilled because it enabled them to easily upcode their billing. He also commented that in his opinion, nothing will make the HIPAA provisions understandable to the general public because they are too complex. He and his colleagues conducted focus groups and tried to explain to people that the health care provider would be responsible for protecting their information with a certain set of exceptions. The response of the focus group participants was to ask if they should trust the health care provider or not. "I do not think readability is going to be the answer with HIPAA," he said. He asked the panelists if they see HIPAA as a barrier to research and as an empowerment for patients.

Ricciardi pointed out that the HHS Office for Civil Rights oversees enforcement of HIPAA and that the HIPAA notice was redrafted 1 year ago with significant input from ONC to be relatively clean, readable, and understandable. She said that she believes the new draft underscores the important point that patients have access to their records and that there are protections in place. Paasche-Orlow responded that he does not think HIPAA is inherently understandable to the patient, to which Ricciardi replied that perhaps it was possible to explain HIPAA generally, albeit not in every detail for every encounter with the health sstem. In response to a comment from Paasche-Orlow that HIPAA seems to be a barrier to the flow of information, Ricciardi added that the sad thing about HIPAA is that it was built with the best intentions and for good reasons, but that it has been implemented terribly. "If we could just get out the word that HIPAA at a minimum guarantees you the right to get your own health information and that you can then share it with anyone you want," said Ricciardi. "I think if that understanding were more prevalent, HIPAA need not be such a barrier to the flow of information."

Rein noted that there is little reason for any institution not to share information with another HIPAA-covered entity, but that is not how the HIPAA regulations are interpreted. She added that there are business interests that exacerbate this problem. She suggested that if the market conditions changed, data liquidity would result. Where she is spending time, she said, is thinking about the non-HIPAA-covered entities, how data are flowing among commercial interests that may not be covered by HIPAA, and what reasonable protections might be. "I think that terrain is wide open for further exploration," said Rein.

The final question in the discussion came from Jennifer Dillaha, who asked the panelists if they were aware of the Family Educational Rights and Privacy Act (FERPA). That Act limits the health care system's access to the tremendous amount of health data in the educational system. Rein said she did not have a solution to this problem and that it was another example of where there are data that have to do with health that are not held by traditional health entities. "It is not until we have a different model of payment where people are actually responsible and accountable for the health of a population that we are going to see data flowing between and across all of those entities because they realize that just doing little things around the 10 percent of your health that is attributable to care does not actually make people healthier," said Rein. She added that in the interim, the federal government has been working over the past 5 or 6 years on open data, establishing plans for exposing more data resources and, hopefully, having greater communication and collaboration among federal agencies. "Maybe there is an opportunity to flag this issue at that level and see if there could be some interim attraction before we have solved the payment reform problem," said Rein. Ricciardi, while acknowledging that she is not a FERPA expert, said she believes FERPA has right-of-access provisions similar to those in HIPAA—that people have a right to their data. "Maybe, just like with Blue Button and health information in general, the individual is part of the solution here," said Ricciardi. "You get your own data and you are able to combine them with data from other sources and share them with whomever you please. I would think about that as a solution—empowering the individual to be the one who gets the data and shares them."

5

Health Information Technology and Selected Populations

The workshop's third and final panel featured three presentations on how thoughtfully designed consumer-facing technologies can be used to reach and improve the health of selected populations. Katherine Kim, assistant professor at the Betty Irene Moore School of Nursing at the University of California, Davis, spoke about the use of consumer-facing technologies with Native American populations. Elizabeth Jordan, associate professor and senior assistant dean of undergraduate nursing at the University of South Florida's College of Nursing, described how mobile technologies can provide critical information that can help pregnant women and new mothers improve their health and the health of their babies. Winston Wong, medical director at Kaiser Permanente discussed the promises and perils of technology that were brought up in an IOM workshop on digital health strategies, health disparities, and health equity conducted by the Roundtable on the Promotion of Health Equity and the Elimination of Health Disparities. An open discussion moderated by Pamela Jeffries followed the presentations.

ISSUES AND USE IN NATIVE AMERICAN POPULATIONS[1]

The message that Katherine Kim said she wanted the workshop participants to take home is that there are types and there are stereotypes. "We

---

[1] This section is based on the presentation by Katherine Kim, assistant professor at the Betty Irene Moore School of Nursing at the University of California, Davis, and the statements are not endorsed or verified by the IOM.

tend to build technology to the stereotypes," she said, and she illustrated this point by referring to herself. "What you probably see in front of you is a middle-aged Asian woman, fairly well educated because you just heard my biography, and I have some technology experience. What you do not know about me that I just learned about myself is that I am 3.4 percent Neanderthal, and when I learned that, it had a huge impact on my perception of my health. I somehow felt more vigorous, more robust, like I could take on anything, which is important because I had gestational diabetes with my second child and have been told that I am at increased risk for developing diabetes, so I should lose some weight."

"The other thing that you should know about me," Kim continued, "is that there is one thing that I do related to my health very actively and very regularly every single day whether I am at home or whether I am traveling, and that is brush my teeth. That is the one point at which you always know I am going to do something about my health." Given that information, she challenged the participants to build an app for her that would help her lose weight. "Had you built from my stereotype, you would have said, 'She does not care so much about weight, is not that concerned about diabetes because Koreans are not in the group of Asians that are prone to diabetes, and probably uses lots of health apps because she is in this field;' but I have no health apps on my phone. You would have built something for someone like me assuming something. Knowing something about me though, you might now build something different."

Turning to the subject of addressing structural health disparities and the digital divide facing Native American populations, Kim explained that there are 3.7 million American Indian and Alaskan Native people in the United States. The Indian Health Service is the primary care provider for 2.2 million of these individuals, most of whom live on reservations. Life expectancy is 4.2 years less than for the rest of the American population and all-cause mortality is 1.2 times higher. Not only are there significant health disparities affecting this population, but there is also a great digital divide. Kim noted that most people want to get health information from the Internet in someplace private, and for most Americans that means having home Internet access. "We know that 96 percent of the richest people in the United States have home Internet and only 25 percent of the poorest," said Kim. Only 30 percent of Native Americans have access to in-home broadband service, which she said is critical for accessing most health information technologies, compared to 69 percent for Asian Americans, who have the highest level of broadband adoption. "When you have broadband, you do different things. You can use sites that have rich and dynamic content. You can look at news. You can search for jobs and submit applications for jobs. You can look at blogs and post blogs, and you can publish your own information," explained Kim. The digital divide extends to schools as well. In schools in which minorities make up the majority of students, there are 37 percent more users per Internet-connected computer.

In this context, said Kim, efforts to address the digital divide among Native Americans has focused on providing access to broadband service in tribal centers and public libraries. She specifically mentioned efforts by The Bill & Melinda Gates Foundation that brought broadband connectivity, hardware, software, training, and education to Native American communities. The federal government's Broadband Technology Opportunity Program is also providing funds to rural communities in general and Native American communities in particular, though this program does not address the "last mile issue," which is getting broadband into the home. Kim called this a critical infrastructure gap. Nonetheless, public and tribal libraries are now providing critical access to health information to Native Americans, and she noted that NLM has a Native American outreach program to create targeted health-related content and to support developing the infrastructure to tribal communities.

Once infrastructure is in place, it is then possible to think about how to use that infrastructure to improve the health of these underserved communities, but as Kim noted, little research has been done on the best way to do so for Native American communities. She referred to a systematic review of the literature on technology and health disparities conducted in 2012 (Montague and Perchonok, 2012) that found only four papers that even mentioned Native Americans. In an update of this review, Kim and her colleagues found two more papers. "There may be things going on in these communities, but they are not in academic publications," said Kim. The published work has focused primarily on online education because the access to K-12 education for tribal communities is still quite limited, she explained.

The Indian Health Service's telemedicine efforts, rather than focusing on consumer-facing technology, have centered mostly on clinic-facing technology that provides access to specialty consults. These efforts have produced good results in terms of wait times for specialty consults and access to specialists that were not available at all prior to telemedicine, Kim explained. She also highlighted the MyPreventiveCare program, which Alex Krist discussed earlier in the workshop, and the Mobile Health for Youth effort. The former provides an interactive preventive health record at practice-based research networks, two of which serve a significant number of Native Americans. The latter focuses on sexually transmitted diseases and teen pregnancy. She said more work is needed in Native American communities and that a couple of the programs discussed at the workshop presented opportunities to do just that using culturally grounded evidence and technology enablement.

To illustrate those opportunities, Kim discussed her own work. With regard to culturally grounded evidence, she took words that represented traditional Native American values (Coyhis and Simonelli, 2008), many of which most investigators would not use in describing their health information technology research, such as patience, balance, humility, spiritual, respect, sovereignty, restitution, autonomy, calmness, and plurality (see Figure 5-1). "It is important that these traditional values actually come throughout the entire continuum of research and development in order for us to really engage the Native American community in improving community health," said Kim. She noted that the National Congress of American Indians (NCAI) developed a research agenda in 2007 that includes addiction and diabetes as two of the health issues in which NCAI was interested. NCAI also developed a tribal research curriculum that was intended to help tribal members engage successfully in research.

In her project, which is funded by the U.S. Department of Agriculture, Kim and her colleagues are working with three tribes in Northern California and Southern Oregon: the Karuk, the Yurok, and the Klamath tribes. The project's goal is to engage tribal youth with mobile technology so that they become the drivers of community health, and one of the tools Kim's team used is a research and leadership development curriculum that engages youth to become community researchers. After several weeks of training, tribal youth were able to design a research project and use mobile technology to conduct the research. Kim noted that four members of the youth research team presented the first results of this project to a packed room of physicians, nurses, researchers, and community members at the University of California, Davis, Clinical Translational Sciences Center. The

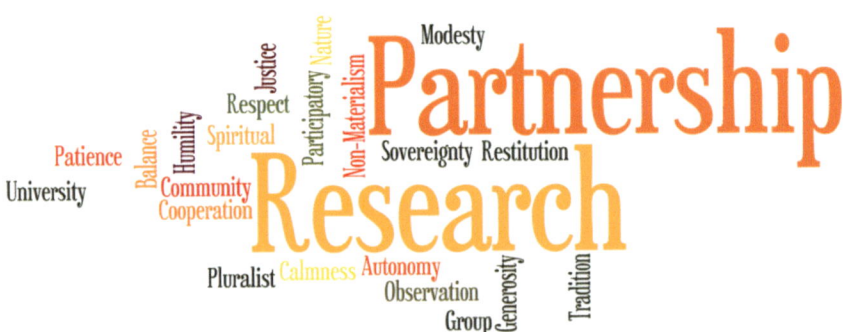

FIGURE 5-1 Words that represent traditional Native American values are a piece of culturally grounded evidence.
SOURCE: Kim presentation, March 24, 2015.

youth researchers gave her permission to discuss the project results at this workshop and have approved the content of this presentation.

The youth researchers first considered four different methodologies that they felt were culturally appropriate because they involved storytelling: survey, interview, graffiti wall, and photo voice. They decided to conduct a community food and health assessment and selected two methodologies, a verbally conducted survey and photos. There is little Internet and cell phone connectivity in this region so they used Magpi software to develop the survey instrument that could be used on their iPods in disconnected mode and then the survey data uploaded back at the tribal computer center. The survey reached 212 tribal members. One of the compelling results focused on confidence around health food choices and its relationship to physical activity. The results showed that the two were strongly related and so the youth researchers decided to do something around physical activity because that had an impact on confidence about food.

Kim and her colleagues suggested that the youth researchers make a game out of their intervention, but the youth researchers said that collaboration, not competition, is a core tribal value. They also said it was important to engage tribal elders and the wisdom they possess, so they came up with a game called walk-about. The game is a mapped walk that takes participants through the community and the countryside, enabling them to look at native plants, to understand their significance to the tribe, how to prepare them for eating or for use as medicine, and where to gather them. "But this is where community engagement is really important because the data you collect when you have a game like this are GPS location, and some of the walks were going to go to sacred and culturally important tribal sites, which should be protected, not shared indiscriminately outside of the tribe," said Kim. In one story relayed to her in explaining this, a location for harvesting mushrooms was made public and outsiders stripped all the mushrooms and sold them at a farmers' market. This was against the local culture in which community members have respect for the Earth's resources and would take only what they could use or share with others in need. "These are the kinds of things that the tribes are concerned about in terms of sovereignty and protection of resources," said Kim. She also noted that because the nearest small grocery store is 15 miles away and the closest large supermarket is 38 miles away, access to historically important tribal foods that are natural and wild in the environment is critical to the tribe.

The last point Kim made is that technology that is enabled and designed with community engagement takes a similar approach to the design of patient-centered technologies. "User centered is really from the external perspective," she said. "I, as a technology developer, think about what you, as a user, need in order to use my product. I, as a provider or health system administrator, think about what you, as the patient, need to engage in the health care system." Empowerment, she explained, is an internal perspective: "What do I, as the user, need from the system in order for me to do the best I can to improve my health or to improve my experience?"

The use of participatory research and participatory design, said Kim, takes that internal perspective and combines with the cultural context of the community to produce the best technology and the best health intervention design. That, she said, is what she meant at the beginning of her presentation when she talked about not turning types into stereotypes, which would produce a one-size-fits-all technology. "We can actually use social and mobile technologies to design experiences that fulfill individual user's needs, preferences, and values," she said in closing.

MOBILE TECHNOLOGIES FOR PREGNANT WOMEN AND NEW MOTHERS[2]

Elizabeth Jordan discussed some of the lessons learned from the national text4baby program as an exemplar for communicating with pregnant women and new mothers. She noted that she came to work with text4baby through her work with the National Healthy Mothers, Healthy Babies Coalition. The coalition wanted a nursing perspective at the table when it began to launch the text4baby program in 2010.

There are many good reasons to develop a text-based mobile app to reach pregnant women. First, 89 percent of young women have cell phones. Some 99 percent of text messages are read, 90 percent within 3 minutes. People of color are more likely to text than their white counterparts, and low-income Americans text more than higher-income adults. Although text-4baby has developed a mobile app, it began as a program to send short text messages to pregnant mothers. Jordan said the evidence she would discuss comes from the text messaging aspect of the program.

Using text messaging to change health-related behaviors is not new. A 2010 meta-analysis and systematic review of text message–based interventions found evidence to support text messaging as a tool for improving behavioral and clinical outcomes for weight loss, smoking cessation, and diabetes management (Cole-Lewis and Kershaw, 2010). Other studies have shown in randomized controlled trials that text messaging can improve influenza vaccination rates among low-income, urban children, adolescents, and pregnant women (Hofstetter et al., 2015; Stockwell et al., 2015), though another randomized controlled trial found that text message prompts were

---

[2] This section is based on the presentation by Elizabeth Jordan, associate professor and senior assistant dean of undergraduate nursing at the University of South Florida College of Nursing, and the statements are not endorsed or verified by the IOM.

not effective at increasing vaccination rates among low-income, urban pregnant women (Moniz et al., 2013). Jordan noted that the *Journal of Health Communications* published a series of articles on the effectiveness of mobile health technologies to change health-related behavior, including two on text4baby (Evans et al., 2012; Parker et al., 2012).

The text4baby program is a free service provided by the nonprofit National Healthy Mothers, Healthy Babies Coalition. It is the largest mobile health initiative. As of March 14, 2015, Jordan said, 800,122 English-speaking women and 46,372 Spanish-speaking women had enrolled. Johnson & Johnson provided the initial funding, but the program now has more than 1,100 sponsors promoting it, including the White House Office of Science and Technology Policy and HHS. The program focuses on delivering messages to pregnant women and mothers with children under age 1 on a range of key topics, including smoking cessation, breastfeeding, health care access, diabetes, nutrition, oral health, immunization, prenatal care, disabilities, family planning, HIV/AIDS prevention, violence prevention, physical activity, safety and injury prevention, mental health, substance abuse prevention, developmental milestones, labor and delivery, car seat safety, safe sleep, and exercise. The goal is to support mothers in achieving key developmental milestones, thus giving their babies the best possible start in life.

Women learn about the program through word of mouth, at a health care provider's office, in a clinic, and even from community workers who help pregnant women and new mothers enroll in text4baby. Signing up for the program is as simple as texting BABY or BEBE to 511411. The mother-to-be or new mother inputs her due date and zip code, then the system sends free tips approximately three times a week throughout pregnancy and until the baby's first birthday. Through text4baby, women can also learn more about certain topics, get support for enrolling in Medicaid or the Children's Health Insurance Program (CHIP), take quizzes, get urgent health alerts, sign up for appointments, receive notifications of the Special Supplemental Nutrition Program for Women, Infants, and Children (WIC) meetings and vaccination reminders, provide feedback on specific messages, and get connected to support hotlines. Jordan said that developing evidence-based content that reflected the latest research on readability and reading level was critical in launching the program. This development was done in close collaboration with CDC and was guided by the mobile health conceptual model of behavior change developed by Douglas Evans (Evans et al., 2012). All content received a rigorous review by a content development council that had representatives from the American Academy of Pediatrics; American College of Nurse-Midwives; American College of Obstetricians and Gynecologists; Association of Women's Health, Obstetric and Neonatal Nurses; CDC; HRSA; March of Dimes; National Association of Pediatric Nurse Practitioners; and the Society for Maternal-Fetal Medicine.

Interactivity is a key feature of the text4baby program. Of the 267 messages that the program sends out, 58 percent contain additional health and resource information, 46 percent contain links to the text4baby mobile webpages developed in partnership with major medical associations, and 25 percent provide a phone number for resources such as local food banks and domestic violence hotlines. There are also 45 links to informational videos and 15 visit and appointment reminders. Nine messages prompt mothers to text back "LIKE" when they find a message helpful, and seven messages encourage mothers to text back "MORE" to get additional information. Quizzes on food safety and pregnancy as well as car seat safety in infancy are also included.

For women with at least a high school education, text4baby showed a positive effect with regard to knowledge that alcohol use will harm a baby and about the value of prenatal vitamins. Nearly two-thirds of new mothers reported that text4baby helped them remember a vaccination appointment, and 74 percent of users reported learning about a medical warning sign, both during their pregnancies and in the newborns. Two-thirds of the users reported talking to a provider about a topic from a text4baby message.

Text4baby, said Jordan, is a data-driven initiative, and staff routinely monitor and analyze a wide array of data collected through the mobile platform and other sources. Aggregate data are available on the text4baby website, and specific data can be accessed upon completion of a data agreement usage form. Available data include enrollment and cancellation data, survey data, and interactive module use. Some anecdotal data obtained from participant feedback phone calls, discussion groups, and social media sites are also available.

As an example of how text4baby works, Jordan discussed the influenza module, which was developed in 2012. "The idea was that we wanted to know if we could improve the rates of flu vaccinations by using messages for pregnant women and moms with infants," she explained, and to overcome various barriers, such as forgetting or getting too busy, the cost of vaccination, and health concerns related to the safety and efficacy of influenza vaccination. On October 15, 2012, all current enrollees, some 89,000 women, were sent the message "Flu season is here and we're checking in with moms. Are you planning to get a flu shot this year?" and 28,609 women responded. Those who responded were asked if they would like a general reminder or something more specific. For those who were not planning on getting a flu shot, the program asked the user why not. A follow-up message was sent on November 27, 2012, asking if the user had gotten a flu shot. For women who identified cost as a barrier, the text4baby program provided a local source for free vaccinations, and these women were two times more likely to get vaccinated. What that shows, said Jordan, is that mobile health apps can overcome barriers and connect women with the care they need.

Jordan also said that text4baby partnered with the Connecting Kids to Coverage initiative of the Centers for Medicare & Medicaid Services to drive enrollment in CHIP, Medicaid, and text4baby. Three days after enrolling in text4baby, the Medicaid module sends a message asking the women about the type of insurance they have. Those who respond that they have no health insurance are sent information on Medicaid/CHIP, with a follow-up message sent 1 week later to see if the women had applied for insurance. Those who respond that they have Medicaid/CHIP or who indicate that they have applied for coverage receive information on how to renew their coverage through these programs, Jordan said.

LESSONS LEARNED FROM THE WORKSHOP ON DIGITAL HEALTH STRATEGIES, HEALTH DISPARITIES, AND HEALTH EQUITY[3]

The workshop's final presentation, delivered by Winston Wong, discussed some of the lessons learned from an IOM Roundtable on Health Equity and the Elimination of Health Disparities meeting that was held in Detroit on October 2, 2014. He noted that the previous two presentations would have fit well in the context of that meeting. He also explained that the meeting was held in Detroit because it has some of the worst health disparities in the United States, particularly with regard to infant mortality.

The focus of that workshop was to explore how communities are using digital health technologies to improve health outcomes for vulnerable population groups and to investigate community engagement efforts to improve access to high-quality health information. The workshop also discussed the need for models of successful technology-based strategies to reduce health disparities. One key theme in the workshop was that digital health strategies have the potential to both exacerbate and diminish already existing disparities among population groups, a point that Wong said was also made at this workshop. Another theme was that addressing health disparities is not about technology, but rather is about people. "Technology is extremely seductive and we are bombarded daily about the promise of technology," said Wong. "But technology should be the servant, not the master." The importance of engaging the community in health behavior change and addressing disparities was another theme that emerged from

---

[3] This section is based on the presentation by Winston Wong, medical director for community benefit disparities improvement and quality initiatives at Kaiser Permanente, and the statements are not endorsed or verified by the IOM.

the Detroit workshop's discussions, as was the need to look at systems and patterns rather than at individual, isolated events.

As was the case at this current workshop, the Detroit workshop made the point that there is already extensive use of mobile technologies in minority communities, particularly among the younger segments of the American population where smartphone use is nearly ubiquitous. As one Detroit workshop participant noted, more people globally own a cell phone than own a toothbrush, and Wong remarked how intriguing it is too see photos of people in the most isolated parts of Africa using their cell phones.

As Kim stressed, community engagement is critical, as is participatory research. Outreach efforts have to be ongoing, said Wong, and there is a need to think about ways to incentivize participation, not in terms of the stereotypes that Kim mentioned, but in terms of what is relevant to specific communities. In that respect, it is essential to align research questions with community and patient needs. The text4baby program, noted Wong, is an example of a program that involves local individuals in efforts to customize messages to reflect community and patient needs.

One speaker at the Detroit workshop said rather provocatively that mobile technology is where it is at, and to demonstrate that notion, the workshop featured lunchtime presentations by producers of different mobile health technologies. "We saw mobile health applications that had to do with connecting people to healthy foods, to WIC vouchers, and other things that were not just about engaging individuals with regard to health behaviors, but also connecting people to resources," said Wong.

Mobile health technology, said Wong, can reduce the digital divide and mobile technology allows for customizing digital health technology. Mobile technology is also useful for centralizing communication and gathering information across people and systems. One mobile health application that was discussed at the earlier workshop could track menstrual cycles for "less risky sex," though one could argue that it could be used to increase fertility, too.

The workshop also highlighted that there are perils associated with digital health technology. Time commitments can cause health care staff to push back against technology adoption, as can the fear that technology will replace personal interactions between providers and patients. Health literacy is also needed to use these tools, and today, little effort is made to evaluate both the usability and utility of these tools, as was also mentioned at this workshop. Toward that end, the Detroit workshop stressed the importance of the technology industry working with members of the health care field, as well as young people, on creating evidence-based apps and other technologies with user-centered designs. In addition, the Detroit workshop noted the lack of diversity in the technology world and questioned how industry would develop technologies for people of different backgrounds and needs without involving individuals from those underrepresented communities in the design process. "This is a question of how do we democratize the development of health technology," said Wong. Another industry-related concern had to do with the disconnect between the technologies that industry is developing with the profit motive in mind and actual needs as far as improved health outcomes.

Other concerns about digital health technology in general include issues of privacy, the volume of material that consumers may need to deal with, and the amount and complexity of that information. A critical question that remains to be answered, said Wong, is determining what works for whom and under what circumstances. One concern that Wong found interesting was about the need to make digital health technologies "hackable," that is, they need to be customizable by the user. This point, he said, was raised by an office of ZeroDivide, a nonprofit organization based in San Francisco that studies ways of overcoming the digital divide among vulnerable populations. ZeroDivide sponsors hack-a-thons for different communities at which community members look at different technologies and alter them to make them more relevant to their needs.

Wong noted that the cost of connectivity is not declining, and access issues remain as serious as ever. "There are certainly issues about reaching people who need to be reached and not necessarily assuming that everybody has access to the Internet," said Wong. He mentioned Kaiser Permanente's HealthConnect system, which is available to every Kaiser member and can provide lab results, enable prescriptions to be refilled, and give users the ability to email their physicians. This system also has the ability to accept digital photos that can be sent to care team members. Wong said that HealthConnect has transformed Kaiser's ability to connect with patients and how the organization thinks about health care delivery. "Indeed, 35 percent of all the interactions that any primary care physician has at Kaiser Permanente are now through email as opposed to face-to-face and telephone visits, which has led to quality improvement in the delivery of care," he said. However, usage is not equitable across all groups and there are Kaiser members who have access, who do not have access but want it, and who do not have access and do not want it.

The moral of the story, said Wong in his concluding remarks, is that digital health technologies have the potential to both exacerbate and diminish already existing disparities among population groups. The main takeaway message, then, is that it is critical to engage the targeted populations in underserved communities. "If we don't engage people in the communities that have historically been underserved, we are not really addressing the issues of health equity," said Wong.

DISCUSSION

Pamela Jeffries started the discussion by asking what could be done to reduce the initial cost of technology, a factor that seems to contribute to health disparities. Kim replied, "Make it cheaper," and she noted that it is not just the cost of the device, but of the data plan, training, and data storage that contribute to the overall cost of technology. One reason why her project used iPods as the base technology was because it does not rely on a data plan or cell phone plan, can be disconnected from the Internet and still used, which keeps the cost down. Her team used the Magpi software package, which was originally created for use by health workers in Africa, because it is free, further reducing the cost of the technology. "You can have the full functionality of a very robust survey interview tool, but it is free and you can customize it to what you need," said Kim. The tribes are now using this software to customize their survey tool for a different purpose in the same project. "Whatever we can do to reduce the ongoing cost and maintenance cost for technologies for underserved communities, we need to explore those options," she said. One advantage of using text messaging, said Jordan, is that it keeps the cost of technology down and can be used with inexpensive regular mobile phones.

Wong wondered if health plans will start looking at their portals to see if there should be a co-payment for access into the portal, just as there are now co-payments for pharmaceuticals. He also noted, though, that some people are arguing that it is a human right now to have access to information as a critical part of maintaining health.

Jeffries then asked the panelists to comment on the challenges of conducting research on these mobile strategies. Jordan said that although the randomized controlled trial has traditionally been considered the best way to conduct research that will produce the strongest science, it is often difficult with mobile technologies to fund these randomized controlled trials and to collect data in real time. "I do think that there is a need for rigorous evaluations that might be in lieu of the randomized controlled trial," she said.

Kim addressed the question by first noting that it is not just health literacy that needs to be accounted for, but also community literacy on the part of the researcher. "We as researchers need to have cultural humility around what we don't know and have some literacy about how to best engage a community if we want these interventions to work in the best way they can," said Kim. Moreover, access to a device is not the only challenge that needs to be overcome. "Every one of these devices and every one of the applications running on those devices has issues with acceptance, usability, and usefulness for our participants," Kim said, adding that without adoption and acceptance, and without working out all of the feasibility issues, there is no sense in even thinking about a randomized controlled trial.

Junyang Wang of FDA asked the panel how they look at subpopulations and minorities when it comes to clinical trials, given that there are only so many subdivisions that can be made before a clinical trial loses its power. "What factors do you think are the really important ones to consider?" he asked. Wong replied that the community is a good level to get to, but having said that, he added that there is a political issue with regard to disaggregation of the racial and ethnic categories commonly used in the United States. He noted that the designations Asian and Pacific Islander, Latino, and African American have limited clinical significance because these groups are so heterogeneous. "I'm not a research scientist so I do not know where the p values start to get diluted, but I think we have to make the commitment to understand in the United States, which probably has the most unique population in the world. We cannot really uncover hidden disparities until we understand the science of disaggregation," said Wong.

Wang then remarked that FDA is now posting demographic information on clinical trials in what is known as the Drug Trial Snapshot as part of the FDA Safety and Innovation Act requirements for including demographic subgroups in clinical trials. He then asked the panel if they had any ideas about how best to communicate that type of nuance to the public. "Will they look at these data in a way that will help them in their medical decisions?" he asked, and if so, does the benefit from using demographic subgroups in clinical trials outweigh the statistical challenge of getting answers from those trials. Kim responded that erring on the side of access to information is better than lack of access simply because of worries about whether people will understand the information. As an example, she cited her experience working with the Karuk tribe youth, who discovered through their participation in this research project just how much their community was concerned about the health of their residents. When these youth saw that issues like obesity were a concern, they were then able to look at national statistics and discover that this is also a national concern and then discuss how important this was to them and what they should do about it. "I think that having some context about what information is available that you can actually use to think about technology and think about health interventions in your community is beneficial to those people trying to make a change," said Kim.

Lindsey Robinson, trustee for the 13th District of the American Dental Association, noted that health disparities also extend to dental health and that 80 percent of the disease burden affects 20 percent of the population. In fact, she said, CDC recently released data showing that there has been a modest improvement in reducing the prevalence of dental caries in young white children, but not in Hispanics and African Americans. In some Native

American tribes, she added, 75 percent of the children under age 3 need to be treated in the operating room because their early childhood caries are so severe. Robinson asked Kim if there was anything about oral health in her project. Kim responded that oral health did not come up in the discussions with the communities she worked with because the focus so far has been on food. "If we had more time to think about other aspects of health disparities, it might have come up, but our role as facilitators was not to push them to think about an issue that we thought was important," said Kim.

Jeffries wondered if those communities even know about the prevalence of oral health problems, and Wong noted that in the Alaskan Native population, the incidence of dental caries has soared over the past two generations. He suggested that embracing the knowledge of elders and their culture could play an important role here, just as it did when developing the walking game in Kim's project.

Gem Daus, public health analyst at HRSA, asked the panelists if they could give specific examples of how digital technologies exacerbate disparities. Wong replied that one place that technology exacerbates disparities is seen in early adopters. "I see it in San Francisco, which is the heart of the digital divide, because you see so many individuals who are invested in their self-fitness and wellness while we have probably the worst homeless population in the country," he said. "There is a divide and an exacerbation with regard to disparities because we see the fallout between people who are really high accelerators and early adopters of self-actualization strategies as opposed to population-level strategies to increase the wealth of health across a different community."

Kim said that a project she recently completed in San Francisco implemented a mobile app for youth with obesity and depression to enable them to do self-tracking, look at their own behavior patterns, and work with a health coach. One of the most striking outcomes is the increase in the levels of patient activation. She thought there were several reasons for this increase in activation. Participants reported, for example, that they had never had a person, the health coach in this case, who just wanted to listen to them. They also reported that it was empowering to be able to look at their own data, decide what they meant, and then decide where they wanted to change if they wanted to change. That is self-efficacy that Kim believes will drive the long-term impact on the health of the participants. Returning to the question of disparities, she said that without the generous support of the Robert Wood Johnson Foundation, which enabled her team to purchase iPods for each participant, this intervention would not have been possible. "This is not something that public health departments can do," she said. "They cannot buy these devices for every young person in San Francisco, so we cannot scale this unless there is a funding source."

Robert Logan noted that large health maintenance organizations have reported more success over time with patient portals and health information technology interventions than any other health care institutions in the United States. He asked Wong for his opinion about whether that success arises because people have to make a commitment to become a member of one of those organizations and, in return, those organizations make a commitment to provide an early return on investment to its members by investing in user-friendly and useful portals and other digital health interventions. Wong replied that the question raised a relevant point and noted that Kaiser Permanente's marketing surveys have found there is a culture of people who will never consider becoming Kaiser members, but that the 30 percent of the public who do become members, and he stressed the word "members," stay with Kaiser Permanente. "People think of their relationship to Kaiser Permanente as a member as opposed to being a patient and as opposed to being a consumer. I think the member affiliation makes it easier to connect to people in terms of why would you want to have reminders, why would you want a health plan to tell you that you should walk or exercise 30 minutes a day," said Wong. He also recounted a recent conversation he had with Kaiser's former chief executive officer, who said that the organization is invested in making sure that its members stay healthy because it does not make money when its members get sick. Wong added that this idea is the foundation on which most of the historic health maintenance organizations were established.

Addressing Kim, Logan said that one of the challenges that NLM finds in working with Native American communities is that many Native Americans live in urban areas now, not on reservations. This is a larger problem, he said, because the health statistics for Native Americans living in urban areas are much worse than for those living on reservations, while at the same time there may be no urban Native American community with which to connect and draw upon when developing or enacting interventions. He then asked Kim how her model works when that sense of community is diluted significantly. Kim began her reply by explaining that her children are actually one-sixteenth Native American, but that they have never identified themselves as Native American on any Census or other survey. "That is often what you see both in the reservation communities and urban communities. Native Americans identify themselves as 'multiple,' which means that you might not even know how many people identify as Native American." The question then becomes one of how to engage a community when neither the boundaries nor the identity of that community are clear, she said.

She then compared the work she and her colleagues have conducted with Klamath Basin youth and urban youth in San Francisco. In this city, the students identified with a school community, not an ethnicity. The connection to a community was absent when she worked with youth through the San Francisco General Family Health Center. "They were the hardest to engage and keep in the intervention because their primary relationship was with a physician they rarely saw," said Kim. The key, she added, is to think about the community that needs to be engaged, not necessarily the ethnic group. "To me, that's a type, not a stereotype. A school is a type of a community, and it is not the stereotype in which every school community is like every other school community," said Kim. The challenge, she added, is to identify the boundaries of each specific community.

A workshop participant then asked the panelists if they had any thoughts about how to convince the private sector that there is something to be done for chronic diseases such as hypertension, diabetes, HIV, renal disease, tuberculosis, and others in underserved populations that do not have money to spend, yet need help the most. Kim, who noted that she has spent most of her career in the private sector before moving back to academia, said the private sector is not necessarily driven by return on investment, but rather by profit, and there is profit to be made in population health. "What the business model is I don't know yet, but there is money to be made in population health because we are all trying to improve population health," Kim said. "There is research money going into that. There is health system money going into that. There is public health department money going into that." She noted that there was a Robert Wood Johnson Foundation Quantified Self Public Health workshop being held in which the conversation was going to be about how to bring those in public health and community health together with technology people and develop a business model that incentivizes companies to take on this mission.

Dean Hovey said the key is to remember that people in the United States want to serve and help. The challenge is to identify those individuals and companies in the private sector and in the foundation sector that care and stimulate their interest and involvement in this area. He noted that the for-profit projects that his company is working on are spilling over into other less profitable applications. He reminded the workshop that Apple was always generous about putting computers into classrooms as a foundation for later business. Wong added that one-third of all Californians are covered under Medicaid today, so by definition that is a low-income group, yet there is money there. He also commented that there are businesses in the retail sector that market specifically to lower-income communities and they have figured out how to be profitable. "I think that there is going to be some segmentation with regards to how technology is starting to be parsed out to different population groups based on their discretionary income, just as there is in retail," said Wong.

As a final comment, Laurie Myers provided a quote from George Merck, the founder of her company, who said, "We try never to forget that medicine is for the people. It is not for the profits. The profits follow, and if we have remembered that, they have never failed to appear. The better we have remembered it, the larger they have been." She recounted this quote to remind workshop participants that no matter where people come from, they still need help, and this community has the responsibility of making sure they get that help. From her perspective as someone who has been thinking about how to apply universal precautions to all of her communications with patients, she said she believes digital health can help with this. The challenge will be for big companies such as hers, where things do not happen fast, to work with small, nimble technology companies to address these needs in a way that benefits the health of the nation sooner rather than later.

6

Reflections on the Day

The workshop's final session focused on reflections on the day's proceedings. Rima Rudd said she was encouraged by the shift in focus from the individual to the community. "Once you are talking about community, the potential for change and action is grand," she said. With asthma, for example, a focus on community starts a conversion on housing stock, air pollution from idling buses, and changing traffic patterns to deal with the larger triggers of asthma in an entire community. Wilma Alvarado-Little echoed those comments and added that one challenge in working with communities is overcoming the suspicion that researchers are going to tell them what they want rather than truly listen and learn about what the community believes it needs. She noted, too, the importance of considering language when working with communities in which English may not be the first language for many community members. "We have to question in what language do they get sick and in what language do they access their emotions," she explained.

Rudd was also buoyed by the fact that there is renewed attention to formative research rigor and to the importance of understanding the people who make up the intended audience before creating an intervention and then iteratively piloting to see how best to produce change with that audience. "We do not allow drugs on the market without that rigor, yet we allow messages and information on the market without rigor," said Rudd. "Information that is not accessible cannot be accessed by anyone."

Stacey Rosen, associate professor of cardiology at Hofstra North Shore–Long Island Jewish (LIJ) School of Medicine and vice president for women's health at the North Shore–LIJ Health System, identified as important the emphasis on creating truly customized approaches to using health information technology to reach specific audiences and the value that each individual gleans from comparing his or her data to that of their community. She also noted the importance of the end users, including patients, care providers, and community members, being involved in the creation of these interventions, as she believes the current state of EHRs is tied to the fact that they were created without this kind of input. Terry Davis reiterated the importance of designing technology in collaboration with the end users, but also pointed out that it still may be necessary to teach people how to use these technologies and to make them more user-friendly.

Christopher Dezii said he got the message that apps are not a panacea, but are merely a tool that may or may not be useful, depending on patient needs. Given that the prevalence and penetration of technology is going to be different 20 years from now than it is today, he believes the field needs to find apps that are successful in today's world, but also prepare for the world 20 years from now, when prices will come down to a point that just about everybody can have whatever his or her children have today. He also felt that the linkage of technologies with providers was another important issue that the field needs to address. Interoperability has to be a key, not just among apps, but among providers. He remarked that he had the sense that health literacy and patient education are still considered a luxury that is always just behind something more important. Changing this attitude will require providers and health care systems to be accountable for health literacy via performance measure development connected to reimbursement policies. He said patient engagement measures need to change from just checking off a box that patients were engaged to determining whether patients understood the information conveyed by their care providers.

Robert Logan concluded from Alex Krist's findings that seniors used the portal he studied more than expected while young adults used it less to mean that socioeconomic characteristics may not predict engagement for sustained use along preconceived lines, raising the question of how best to develop the conceptual framework for evaluation metrics. Inclusion of health literacy as a conceptual framework and its inclusion as part of the evaluation instrument might help to better predict patient engagement, sustained use, and other desirable outcomes, he said. He also remarked that roundtable discussions could be helpful in demonstrating how the addition of health literacy is useful conceptually in app and website development, that it contributes to better understanding of intended users, and that the addition of health literacy as a measure is a useful component for evaluating patient portals, health apps, and health literacy websites.

Terri Ann Parnell, principal and founder of Health Literacy Partners, applauded the speakers on the third panel for the work they were doing, saying that, in her opinion, they have demonstrated that access is a central issue that needs to be addressed. She also took away from these presentations the idea that trust, face-to-face communications, building relationships, and community engagement are critical to the success of digital health technology. "We need to bring together the patient or the consumer along with the professional and community along the journey so that we have a product that is useful and meaningful to all," said Parnell. Even with easy access, a technology that is not meaningful to the users will not be used. Michael Villaire, however, said he is very concerned about the issue of access and the disparities between those who can get and use these applications and those who cannot.

Laurie Myers said she wanted to reiterate the importance of the system factors in facilitating the adoption of health technology. Taking a team approach is critical, and the challenge is to figure out how to take advantage of teams to help address and reduce health disparities. "Some of the evolving payment models may help with that," said Myers. Incorporating the new types of data that will be available into workflow and making them actionable will be a challenge that will likely require the development of filters to sort out the data that can actually help improve patient care. Also needed will be the evidence showing that these data lead to improvements in quality and patient outcomes. She applauded the job that the panelists did in talking about the importance of community-based participatory research and said that she believes there are probably lessons from the gaming industry that the field can learn with regard to stickiness and simplicity. Myers also noted the importance of aligning incentives to things that are important to the end users.

Lori Hall, a health education consultant to Eli Lilly, noted how the day's presentations changed her perception that most health information technology interventions were aimed at people who are already engaged, activated, and confident in their care. She now understands that technology developers first seek to understand and listen before making assumptions, and when used in partnership, technology is a tool that can address the needs of communities that are not as engaged in their health care. "Ultimately, this is a statement about technology being important, but that it will never replace empathy," said Hall. Earnestine Willis voiced the same optimism. She reiterated that the message she got from the presentations is that any technology must be relevant to a specific population and it must avoid being designed to serve stereotypes. "We tend to want to say we must make the community fit into our randomized controlled trial box, but I would say this is an opportunity for us to come up with new methods, new analyses, and new methodologies that we can use to begin to get a better picture of these communities." She also noted that taking the opportunity to learn about targeted communities creates the chance to tap into the creativity in these communities to develop novel approaches to increasing health literacy and community health.

Marin Allen, deputy associate director in the Office of Communications and Public Liaison, and director of public information in the Office of the NIH Director, remarked that something magical happened over the course of the day, and she credited Kim. "What she did for us is exactly what Dean Hovey started out with; she created the story arc that I would guess is the one we will find most memorable from this meeting," said Allen. She also commented to Winston Wong that it is necessary to look at resilience as well as disparity to tease out the effects of aggregation about which he voiced concern. As a final comment, she said it is important to start thinking about what communication means in all of its nuances.

Villaire thanked the afternoon panels for showing examples of how to design appropriate and useful technologies and hoped that some of these things can be replicated in other communities. He then said he believes the issue of mobile health technology juxtaposed with health literacy is one of context. "How do we as some of the experts in the area of health literacy provide our expertise to provide context for the information that is being developed?" he asked, particularly as the population's familiarity and comfort with technology changes in the years ahead. He predicted there will be a shift from today's situation in which both researchers and consumers are trying to catch up with the technology to one in which developers will be trying to catch up to those who are using technology. "I'm hoping that these digital users become more demanding of what they are asking from technology," said Villaire. He hopes that in the future, end users would be demanding context for information, not just data, and stated his opinion that "it is our role to act as influencers and mediators in this area to be more demanding and make sure people not only understand these devices or technology, but are able to take that information and apply it, which is our definition of health literacy."

He also responded to a comment made earlier in the day about developers winning contests and then moving on to develop the next app. "Maybe what we need to do is incentivize the developers to go that step further and say you will be rewarded on some kind of whatever the basis is, a commissioned basis or whatever, to the extent that these apps and these technologies start showing results," said Villaire. He added that part of the responsibility of a technology developer is to take that next step and find out whether these are tools that people can understand and use to improve their health.

Margaret Loveland, senior director of global medical affairs at Merck, commented on the importance of attending to privacy concerns given that many of the members of these culturally diverse and economically disadvantaged communities have trust issues. "If we do not address this privacy issue so that they can feel confident, especially when we were talking about the apps and how their information gets transmitted, they are not going to be using them," said Loveland. Today, the majority of people use apps to gain information and they do not expect that their information is going to be delivered to anyone else, she explained. She also remarked that the apps themselves can create new communities if they are well designed.

Gem Daus commented that there are two aphorisms that he has been thinking about: If all you have is a hammer, every problem is a nail, and information in and of itself does not change behavior. The presentations made him think of a corollary, which is that technology in and of itself does not change behavior. "We need things like community, and listening, and to connect investment with some measure of outcomes so that we are not just fascinated by these new toys," said Daus.

Although apps and other health technologies need to be simpler for the patient and consumer to use, Kim Parson, strategic consultant on Proactive Care Strategies for Humana, said they will have greater value if they are also easy for members of the care team to use. To have a large impact, these technologies need to get rid of the noise for the physician and move away from just providing data, to a place where they can help set goals for the patient's health, said Parson. The ultimate value of health literate technology, she added, comes when it connects the patient and all the members of the patient's health care team. "When it can be truly connected, then it can be actionable and valuable to all of us," said Parson.

During the course of the presentations, Lindsey Robinson was wondering where her stakeholder group, those concerned with oral health, fits into this conversation about technology. But she came to realize that it fits in everywhere given its role in diabetes, obesity, cardiac disease, and pregnancy. "I would hope that somewhere in the conversation, oral health would be a component of understanding the impact in all those conditions," she said. In particular, she came back to the statement that only 10 percent of health is related to health care and commented that the best way to impact and improve oral health is through conversations in communities, and imbuing cultures with the understanding of how important oral health is to overall health. In so many cultures, she noted, there is little understanding of this connection or of the fact that tooth decay is not inevitable and that they do not have to suffer the same fate as their parents, who may have lost all of the teeth by the time they were 25 years old. She implored the audience to include oral health in any program, including those such as text4baby, designed to improve a population's overall health.

Suzanne Bakken said she was taken by the notion of a learning health system—not a learning health care system—that includes consumer-generated data. From that perspective, it is important to create a fabric of trust for the digital infrastructure in a learning health system that encourages consumers to both contribute and use data. In that respect, it is essential to make sure that the terms of agreement truly inform consumers about how their data are being used and whether those uses are for a social good or for commercial gain. "People need to be aware of those choices," said Bakken, who said she wanted to see the roundtable apply its expertise on health literacy to learn about and share new approaches that can help consumers really know what they are getting into when they contribute their data as a vital part of a learning health system and so they can do so willingly and with trust in the system.

Winston Wong, noting that the day was both informative and dense with information, described a taxonomy for defining populations that he constructed to help him deal with all of these ideas. Patients form the first level of this taxonomy, and patients can be categorized as individuals with an acute problem, individuals with a chronic problem, and individuals with some sort of maintenance of health or some sort of malady. "I think you have to look at each one of those aspects of being a patient differently in terms of how to construct a health literacy strategy," said Wong. Consumers make up the second level given that consumers have distinctly different expectations than do patients, and members represent the third level. "I think a member connotation is different than a consumer and patient because members expect something with regard to how they interface with what whichever entity they belong," said Wong. The fourth level is community and how technology can be used to facilitate the kind of interactions and engagement between the health system and a given community. When thinking about health literacy, he explained, "It behooves the producers of health technology, as well as the individuals on the health care team and the spectrum of health care providers that extends beyond the walls of the clinic, to consider the operational and critical elements that we have cultivated in our understanding of health literacy." Health literacy, he concluded, becomes a critical strategy that is implemented at every one of these different levels of engagement among patient, consumer, members, and community. "I think we need some work to figure out what are the critical features of health literacy as we think about how we move forward in all of these different parts of the engagement hierarchy," said Wong.

Alicia Fernandez said she was struck by two things. One was how embryonic this field is, with so little known about what works and what does not work. The second was the next topic for conversation should be about levers, for she fears that many of the health technologies discussed over the course of the day are ripe for market failure. As an example, she noted that she recently tried to find a very simple cell phone for her mother, who is starting to experience cognitive difficulties. She was willing to pay any price for such a device, but she could not find one. "It was in that way a complete market failure even though there must be millions of people like my mother who would need a product like that," said Fernandez. What she wants to hear, then, is about the levers that government and health systems and organized medicine and others can use in terms of clarity of standards, ethics, privacy, and other concerns. This would help developers create technologies that are needed and useful.

Steven Rush, director of the Health Literacy Innovations Program at UnitedHealth Group, commented on how this workshop reinforced some of the thoughts he has had about health literacy and technology. It also opened his eyes to a number of issues. One has to do with the number of health-related apps available. "If we think about health literacy as something that is accessible, accurate, understandable, and easy to use and we apply that to what we talked about today, which of the 40,000 to 50,000 apps out there are good? I think that is something that we may want to think about," said Rush, referring to the accuracy and usability of these apps. He applauded the emphasis that the day's presentations placed on including community, together with patients, consumers, and providers, in the technology development process, and he pointed out that consumers may not be able to understand the burden of using a particular app or they may not understand that an app may not produce data that can actually help them better manage their health. He also underscored the issue of sustainability and the importance of person-to-person interactions that can reinforce the value of using a particular app.

Catina O'Leary noted the high level of energy that the presentations and discussions had generated, and the incredible diversity of the technologies that are being developed and deployed to help a wide range of audiences better manage their health. She believes this bodes well for the future. One challenge, she said, is helping people select the best or necessary option from among all the choices they have for the particular context in which they want to use a particular app, wearable device, or website. "These are higher order cognitive decisions that not everybody is equipped to make on their own without help, so who are the helpers?" she asked. One possibility she noted is to draw upon the expertise of community health workers, who she believes are poised to help with some training. She also appealed to the developers in the crowd to think about an app that would help consumers manage their health insurance in the context of their health.

The importance of community was also stressed by Jennifer Dillaha, particularly with regard to reaching those people who truly struggle with low health literacy and with interacting with and navigating the health system. "It becomes incumbent on the health system to provide navigation, care coordination, and case management—that flip side of health literacy," said Dillaha. She also said that the health system is going to have to reconfigure itself to help patients and consumers deal with the data that these new technologies will generate. "There are going to be many people who cannot use their patient portals," she said, "and to have a system that is truly person-centric, we will have to reconfigure ourselves." Relying on community will be one way to accomplish that task, she noted.

Michael Paasche-Orlow supported the call he heard in several presentations for participatory evaluation and research from the beginning through the end of a project. He suggested that health literacy could be a fulcrum for building and assessing these systems. He agreed with Fernandez's worry about market failure, but noted that "the market will take care of the digerati. The question is, how do we as a group call the market to take care of the vulnerable population?" said Paasche-Orlow. He also agreed with Wong's notion of a taxonomy, but was of the opinion that it was a nice way of saying that too many of these apps are rudimentary and are reacting to situations rather than asking how patient-centered health information technology can be created that meets the real needs of patients and consumers.

Linda Harris remarked that while most of the presentations over the course of the day were about apps, she wanted to recount one story of a system that has gone far beyond apps. The U.S. Department of Veterans Affairs (VA), she said, has a program that it started in Florida in which a social worker and a provider go into the home of the most vulnerable veterans, those without much education or income, most of whom are retired. The social worker and provider do an assessment of that family's situation and then bring in a simple, text-based phone system that the patient or family member can use to alert the case worker that there is a problem, such as when a patient has reached a particular pain threshold. In that case, as soon as the case worker receives that text, a message would go out to a pharmacy in the patient's community and a pharmacist would be dispatched to the patient's home. What is nice about this system, said Harris, is that it is patient driven, data driven, and outcomes driven, and in fact, the VA has shown that this system dramatically reduced unnecessary hospitalizations. Harris noted that the VA has now expanded this system nationwide. What this example demonstrates, said Harris in concluding the discussion session, is that improving care is not just about apps, but rather is about creating technology that is patient driven and that lets a patient be a partner in his or her own care.

References

Anderson, G. 2010. *Chronic care: Making the case for ongoing care.* Princeton, NJ: Robert Wood Johnson Foundation. http://www.rwjf.org/en/library/research/2010/01/chronic-care.html (accessed April 1, 2015).

Arcia, A., M. Velez, and S. Bakken. 2015. Style guide: An interdisciplinary communication tool to support the process of generating tailored infographics from electronic health data using ENTICE3. *EGEMS (Washington, DC)* 3(1):1120.

Bodenheimer, T., E. Chen, and H. D. Bennett. 2009. Confronting the growing burden of chronic disease: Can the U.S. health care workforce do the job? *Health Affairs (Millwood)* 28(1):64-74.

Broderick, J., T. Devine, E. Langhans, A. J. Lemerise, S. Lier, and L. Harris. 2014. *Designing health literate mobile apps.* Discussion Paper, Institute of Medicine, Washington, DC.

Cole-Lewis, H., and T. Kershaw. 2010. Text messaging as a tool for behavior change in disease prevention and management. *Epidemiologic Reviews* 32:56-69.

Coyhis, D., and R. Simonelli. 2008. The Native American healing experience. *Substance Use & Misuse* 43(12-13):1927-1949.

Derring, M. J. 2013. *Issue brief: Patient-generated health data and health IT.* U.S. Department of Health and Human Services. https://www.healthit.gov/sites/default/files/pghd_brief_final122013.pdf (accessed April 5, 2015).

Dykes, P. 2015. Consumer-generated health information: Provider "readiness," attitudes, and skills. PowerPoint presentation, Workshop on Consumer-Facing Technology, Institute of Medicine. Washington, DC. March 24, 2015.

Evans, W. D., L. C. Abroms, R. Poropatich, P. E. Nielsen, and J. L. Wallace. 2012. Mobile health evaluation methods: The text4baby case study. *Journal of Health Communication* 17(Suppl 1):22-29.

Fox, S., and M. Duggan. 2012. *Mobile health 2012.* Washington, DC: Pew Research Center.

Fox, S., and M. Duggan. 2013. *Tracking for health.* Washington, DC: Pew Research Center.

Gartner, J.R. and Granter, R.vd M. 2014. Gartner says in 2015, 50 percent of people considering buying a smart wristband will choose a smartwatch instead. Press release. Stamford, CT. http://www.gartner.com/newsroom/id/2913318 (accessed April 1, 2015).

Hibbard, J. H., and J. Greene. 2013. What the evidence shows about patient activation: Better health outcomes and care experiences; fewer data on costs. *Health Affairs (Millwood)* 32(2):207-214.

Hibbard, J., and K. Lorig. 2012. The do's and don'ts of patient engagement in busy office practices. *Journal of Ambulatory Care Management* 35(2):129-132.

Hibbard, J. H., J. Greene, and M. Tusler. 2009. Improving the outcomes of disease management by tailoring care to the patient's level of activation. *American Journal of Managed Care* 15(6):353-360.

Hibbard, J. H., J. Greene, Y. Shi, J. Mittler, and D. Scanlon. 2015. Taking the long view: How well do patient activation scores predict outcomes four years later? *Medical Care Research and Review* 72(3):324-337.

Hofstetter, A. M., C. Y. Vargas, S. Camargo, S. Holleran, D. K. Vawdrey, E. O. Kharbanda, and M. S. Stockwell. 2015. Impacting delayed pediatric influenza vaccination: A randomized controlled trial of text message reminders. *American Journal of Preventive Medicine* 48(4):392-401.

Kim, K. 2015. IT issues and use in Native American populations. PowerPoint presentation, Workshop on Consumer-Facing Technology, Institute of Medicine. Washington, DC. March 24, 2015.

Krist, A. H., R. A. Aycock, R. S. Etz, J. E. Devoe, R. T. Sabo, R. Williams, K. L. Stein, G. Iwamoto, J. Puro, J. Deshazo, P. L. Kashiri, J. Arkind, C. Romney, M. Kano, C. Nelson, D. R. Longo, S. Wolver, and S. H. Woolf. 2014. MyPreventiveCare: Implementation and dissemination of an interactive preventive health record in three practice-based research networks serving disadvantaged patients—a randomized cluster trial. *Implementation Science* 9(1):181.

LeBlanc, T. W., A. L. Back, M. Danis, and A. P. Abernethy. 2014. Electronic health records (EHRs) in the oncology clinic: How clinician interaction with EHRs can improve communication with the patient. *Journal of Oncology Practice* 10(5):317-321.

Ledger, D., and D. McCaffrey. 2014. *Inside wearables: How the science of human behavior change offers the secret to long-term engagement.* Cambridge, MA: Endeavour Partners.

Moniz, M. H., S. Hasley, L. A. Meyn, and R. H. Beigi. 2013. Improving influenza vaccination rates in pregnancy through text messaging: A randomized controlled trial. *Obstetrics & Gynecology* 121(4):734-740.

Montague, E., and J. Perchonok. 2012. Health and wellness technology use by historically underserved health consumers: Systematic review. *Journal of Medical Internet Research* 14(3):e78.

Parker, R. M., E. Dmitrieva, S. Frolov, and J. A. Gazmararian. 2012. Text4baby in the United States and Russia: An opportunity for understanding how mHealth affects maternal and child health. *Journal of Health Communication* 17(Suppl 1):30-36.

PricewaterhouseCoopers. 2014. Healthcare delivery of the future: How digital technology can bridge time and distance between clinicians and consumers. http://www.pwc.se/sv/halso-sjukvard/assets/healthcare-delivery-of-the-future.pdf (accessed April 5, 2015).

Schnall, R. 2015. Design specifications for apps: A case study. PowerPoint presentation, Workshop on Consumer-Facing Technology, Institute of Medicine. Washington, DC. March 24, 2015.

Schnall, R., and S. J. Iribarren. 2015. Review and analysis of existing mobile phone applications for health care-associated infection prevention. *American Journal of Infection Control* 43(6):572-576.

Schnall, R., J. Travers, M. Rojas, and A. Carballo-Dieguez. 2014. eHealth interventions for HIV prevention in high-risk men who have sex with men: A systematic review. *Journal of Medical Internet Research* 16(5):e134.

Seligman, M. 2012. *Flourish.* New York: Free Press.

Stockwell, M. S., A. M. Hofstetter, N. DuRivage, A. Barrett, N. Fernandez, C. Y. Vargas, and S. Camargo. 2015. Text message reminders for second dose of influenza vaccine: A randomized controlled trial. *Pediatrics* 135(1):e83-e91.

Turvey, C., D. Klein, G. Fix, T. P. Hogan, S. Woods, S. R. Simon, M. Charlton, M. Vaughan-Sarrazin, D. M. Zulman, L. Dindo, B. Wakefield, G. Graham, and K. Nazi. 2014. Blue button use by patients to access and share health record information using the Department of Veterans Affairs' online patient portal. *Journal of the American Medical Informatics Association* 21(4):657-663.

Wachter, R. M. 2015. Why health care tech is still so bad. *The New York Times*, March 22, 2015.

The White House. 2012. *Digital government: Building a 21st century platform to better serve the American people*. Washington, DC: The White House.

Appendix A

Workshop Agenda

Consumer-Facing Technology: A Workshop
National Academy of Sciences

National Academy of Sciences Building
2101 Constitution Avenue
Washington, DC

March 24, 2015

8:30 a.m.–8:45	Welcome and Introduction *Bernard Rosof, M.D., Roundtable Chair, Quality in Healthcare Advisory Group*
8:45–9:10	Overview: Consumer-Facing Technology: What Is It and What Are the Issues? *Ted Vickey, M.B.S., FitWell, LLC*
9:10–9:30	Discussion
9:30–10:20	Panel 1: Health Literate Digital Design and Strategies
9:30–9:35	Introduction of Panelists Moderator: *Suzanne Bakken, Ph.D., RN, Columbia University School of Nursing*
9:35–9:50	Design Specifications for Apps: A Case Study *Rebecca Schnall, Ph.D., Columbia University School of Nursing*

9:50-10:05	The Federal Digital Strategy and Health Literacy: How HHS Is Integrating Health Literacy Principles into the Federal Digital Strategy *Read Holman, M.P.H., Program Director and Senior Advisor on Internal Entrepreneurship, HHS IDEA Lab/Office of the Chief Technology Officer, HHS*
10:05-10:20	Patient Portals *Alex Krist, M.D., Virginia Commonwealth University*
10:20-10:35	Break
10:35-10:40	Introduction of Reactor Panel *Susan Bakken, Ph.D., RN*

10:40-11:00	Reactors (5 minutes each)
	    Industry: *Dean Hovey, M.S., Digifit*
	    Foundation: *Catina O'Leary, Ph.D., Health Literacy Missouri*
	    Government: *Lana Moriarty, Office of the National Coordinator*

11:00-11:30	Q & A: All Panelists (Design and Reactor) Moderator: *Suzanne Bakken, Ph.D., RN*
11:30-12:00 p.m.	General Discussion: Q & A from Audience Moderator: *Bernard Rosof, M.D.*
12:00-1:00	Lunch
1:00-2:45	**Panel 2: Catalyzing Widespread Informed Engagement**
1:00-1:05	Introduction of Panelists Moderator: *Bernard Rosof, M.D.*
1:05-1:20	Health Professionals: What Skills Are Needed to Interface with Consumers Around Consumer-Generated Information? *Patricia Dykes, Ph.D., M.A., RN, Partners Health Care*

	1:20-1:35	Incentives for Consumer Engagement *Lygeia Ricciardi, Ed.M., Clear Voice Consulting, LLC*
	1:35-1:50	Ethical, Legal, and Social Issues *Alison Rein, M.S., AcademyHealth*
	1:50-2:15	Q & A for Panel Moderator: *Bernard Rosof, M.D.*
	2:15-2:45	General Discussion and Questions Moderator: *Bernard Rosof, M.D.*
2:45-3:00		Break
3:00-4:30		Panel 3: Health IT and Selected Populations
	3:00-3:05	Introduction of Panelists Moderator: *Pamela Jeffries, Ph.D., RN, Johns Hopkins University School of Nursing*
	3:05-3:20	Issues and Use in Native American Populations *Katherine Kim, Ph.D., University of California, Davis, School of Nursing*
	3:20-3:35	Mobile Technologies for Pregnant Women and New Mothers *Elizabeth Jordan, D.N.Sc., University of South Florida College of Nursing*
	3:35-3:50	Lessons Learned from the Workshop: Digital Health Strategies, Health Disparities, and Health Equity: The Promises and Perils of Technology *Winston Wong, M.D., Kaiser Permanente*
	3:50-4:15	Q & A: Need to Develop the Questions via Email Moderator: *Pamela Jeffries, Ph.D., RN*
4:15-4:45		General Discussion Moderator: *Bernard Rosof, M.D.*

4:45-5:30	Reflections on the Day: Roundtable Members Identify Key Lessons Learned from Workshop
5:30	Adjourn

Appendix B

Biographical Sketches of Workshop Speakers

Patricia Dykes, Ph.D., M.A., RN, FAAN, FACMI, is senior nurse scientist and program director for research in the Center for Patient Safety Research and Practice and the Center for Nursing Excellence at Brigham and Women's Hospital (BWH) and assistant professor at Harvard Medical School, where she has a program of informatics and patient safety research. Dr. Dykes and her team were funded by the Robert Wood Johnson Foundation to develop and test a Web-based fall prevention toolkit. The toolkit was found to significantly reduce falls in acute care hospitals and the results of their study were published in the *Journal of the American Medical Association.* Dr. Dykes and her team have expanded this research and are exploring the use of technology to provide the core set of information needed by care team members (including patients) at the bedside to provide and engage in safe patient care. Dr. Dykes is currently the Partner's health care site principal investigator for a Patient-Centered Outcomes Research Institute (PCORI) and the National Institute on Aging–funded fall prevention clinical trial. She is the author of 2 books and more than 70 peer-reviewed publications and has presented her work related to nursing informatics, clinical documentation, and patient safety both nationally and internationally. She is a member of the National Institutes of Health Biomedical Computing and Health Informatics Study Section, Center for Scientific Review, and an elected Fellow of the American Academy of Nursing and the American College of Medical Informatics.

Read Holman, M.P.H., is a program director in the U.S. Department of Health and Human Services (HHS) Innovation, Design, Entrepreneurship and Action (IDEA) Lab and senior advisor on internal entrepreneurship to the chief technology officer. His focus is on the development of programs and services that promote the use of start-up methodologies as a means to deliberately disrupt and improve government operations and services. Among his portfolio of activities, Mr. Holman manages the HHS Ignite Accelerator and the HHS Ventures Fund.

Prior to the IDEA Lab, Mr. Holman directed the digital strategy of the Center for Medicare & Medicaid Innovation and served in public affairs within the Office of the Secretary, where he bridged the worlds of communications, policy, and Web technologies. Mr. Holman has a B.S. in Biology and an M.P.H. in Health Care Policy and Management.

Dean Hovey, M.S., has started numerous high-tech companies over the past 30 years from his base in Silicon Valley. He is known for his creativity, product design acumen, and customer insights for having co-founded IDEO and for his early work designing the mouse for Apple Computer. His roles span senior executive positions in public companies, as a venture capital general partner, and CEO/founder/entrepreneur. Mr. Hovey received his B.S./M.S. in General Engineering, Product Design from Stanford University.

Pamela R. Jeffries, Ph.D., M.S.N., RN, FAAN, ANEF, vice provost for digital initiatives at Johns Hopkins University and professor at the School of Nursing, is nationally known for her research and work in developing simulations and online teaching and learning. She is well regarded for her expertise in experiential learning, innovative teaching strategies, new pedagogies, and the delivery of content using technology in nursing education. Additionally, Dr. Jeffries is the past president of the interprofessional, international Society for Simulation in Healthcare and a member of the Institute of Medicine's Global Intraprofessional Education Forum, among many other organizations. Dr. Jeffries was newly inducted into the prestigious Sigma Theta Tau Research Hall of Fame and is the recipient of several teaching and research awards from the Midwest Nursing Research Society and the International Nursing Association of Clinical Simulations and Learning, and teaching awards from the National League of Nursing, Sigma Theta Tau, International, and most recently, the American Association of Colleges of Nursing Scholarship of Teaching and Learning Excellence award. She has a B.S.N. from Ball State University and an M.S.N. and a Ph.D. in Nursing from Indiana University.

Elizabeth "Betty" T. Jordan, D.N.Sc., RNC, FAAN, has more than 30 years of clinical experience and significant research expertise in labor and delivery. Dr. Jordan is a recognized international nursing leader in maternal and newborn outcomes research, education, and practice. She is an associate professor and senior assistant dean of undergraduate nursing at the College of Nursing at the University of South Florida. She previously served as the co-director of the Johns Hopkins University Global mHealth Initiative and director of the Johns Hopkins University School of Nursing baccalaureate program.

Dr. Jordan currently serves as program evaluation consultant for the national Text4Baby program. Healthy Mothers, Healthy Babies Coalition launched this domestic mHealth program in 2010. Dr. Jordan serves on the editorial board and as an author for the Association of Women's Health, Obstetric and Neonatal Nurses' (AWHONN's) consumer magazine and website "Healthy Mom & Baby." She has extensive publications in peer-reviewed journals and has made presentations at regional, national, and international conferences. She served on the Board of Directors of AWHONN and the Board for the Healthy Mothers, Healthy Babies Coalition. She was recognized as 1 of the "Top 100 Women in Maryland" for her dedication and service to Maryland in helping address the issue of poor birth outcomes.

Katherine Kim, Ph.D., M.P.H., M.B.A., is an assistant professor at the Betty Irene Moore School of Nursing at the University of California, Davis (UC Davis). Her research focuses on information technology to improve community health, care coordination, and clinical research. Dr. Kim has led research projects using participatory methods to design, implement, and evaluate mobile and social technology–enabled health interventions and distributed research networks. Her areas of clinical interest include cancer, obesity, heart disease, and other chronic conditions. Her work has been funded by the Robert Wood Johnson Foundation, Agency for Healthcare Research and Quality, PCORI, McKesson Foundation, and Boston University National Cancer Institute.

Currently, Dr. Kim leads a research project at the School of Nursing exploring the use of a social networking platform in cancer care and its impact on care. She also conducts research as part of the UC Davis team contributing to a University of California–wide project exploring the connectivity of 3 networks serving more than 21 million patients. The project is funded by a nearly $7 million grant from PCORI, which supports development of a nationwide clinical research network.

Her work has been published in journals such as *Medical Care*, *Journal of the American Medical Association*, and *Nursing Outlook*. She has received best paper nominations from AcademyHealth and the American Medical Informatics Association. Dr. Kim also serves on advisory boards and task forces for iDASH, a National Institutes of Health National Center for Biomedical Computing, the federal Office of the National Coordinator for Health Information Technology, and PCORI.

Prior to her 2014 appointment as an assistant professor at the nursing school, Dr. Kim was the first graduate of the doctoral Nursing Science and Health-Care Leadership program. Over the course of her 4 years in the doctoral program, she was recognized several times for her leadership in the health technology fields. She co-founded the Interprofessional Health Informatics Student Special Interest Group and received a number of scholarships. Previously, Dr. Kim was a professor at San Francisco State University's Health Equity Institute. For more than 20 years, she has led teams to innovate and excel in hospitals and medical groups. She is also an entrepreneur, serving as CEO of a venture-funded start-up, leader of a business incubator, and founder and president of Kim Consultants. She received a B.A. in Biology from Harvard College and an M.P.H. and an M.B.A. from UC Berkeley.

Alex Krist, M.D., M.P.H., is an associate professor of family medicine and population health at Virginia Commonwealth University and active clinician and teacher at the Fairfax Family Practice residency program. He is co-director of the Virginia Ambulatory Care Outcomes Research Network and director of community-engaged research at the Center for Clinical and Translational Research. Dr. Krist's research focuses on implementation of preventive recommendations, patient-centered care, shared decision making, cancer screening, and health information technology.

Lana Moriarty, M.P.H., is acting director for Consumer eHealth in the HHS Office of the National Coordinator's Office of Programs & Engagement. Previously she managed part of the National Health Service Corps (NHSC) and the NURSE Corps programs for the Health Resources and Services Administration (HRSA). She supported participants of the NHSC and NURSE Corps, which delivered care to underserved communities. She also worked with the World Bank Group, ensuring the needs of women and girls were included in the Bank's many overseas development operations.

Catina O'Leary, Ph.D., LMSW, serves as president and CEO of Health Literacy Missouri (HLM). Under her direction, HLM's service network has expanded to include some of the largest employers in Missouri, including pharmaceutical companies, hospital systems, business coalitions, and community-based organizations. Chosen by the *St. Louis Business Journal* for professional excellence and dedication to the community, Dr. O'Leary is a member of the 2013 class of "40 Under 40" leaders. She was recently selected to join FOCUS St. Louis' 39th Leadership St. Louis class. Before her appointment as CEO of HLM, Dr. O'Leary was a faculty member at Washington University School of Medicine in the Department of Psychiatry and the Program on Occupational Therapy. At Washington University, her community-engaged research centered on methods to engage underserved populations in health and social service programs. She focused specifically on women's health.

Dr. O'Leary is the past president and continues to serve on the board of The Bridge, a drop-in shelter that offers daily meals and basic social services to homeless and at-risk St. Louisans. She also serves as vice president for Magdalene St. Louis, a nonprofit that helps women who have survived lives of abuse, prostitution, trafficking, and addiction by providing a community where they can recover and rebuild their lives.

Dr. O'Leary earned her B.A. in Psychology from the University of Mississippi and an M.S.W. and a Ph.D. in Social Work from the George Warren Brown School of Social Work at Washington University.

Alison Rein is a senior director for evidence generation and translation at AcademyHealth, where she oversees a portfolio that investigates how new sources of data and expanded stakeholder engagement are helping to transform health care and research. Ms. Rein is the principal investigator on a PCORI contract that actively manages and facilitates collaboration among 50 pilot projects to advance the field of patient-centered outcomes research (PCOR), and co-investigator on the Electronic Data Methods Forum. She also recently directed the Beacon Evidence and Innovation Network, which provided Beacon Community Cooperative Agreement Program participants in identifying, documenting, and disseminating the lessons and results of their individual efforts in a systematic way. Ms. Rein serves as AcademyHealth's liaison to the innovations and "open health data" movement spearheaded by HHS, and oversees or contributes to projects that focus on building infrastructure to support quality improvement, comparative effectiveness research, and PCOR.

Ms. Rein has expertise in health information technology policy, stakeholder engagement, comparative effectiveness research, information management and governance, and community-based quality improvement, and has written and presented on a number of these topics. With more than 18 years of experience in the health care field, she brings a range of skills to her work, including technical assistance design and execution, collaborative network development, research design, and policy analysis.

Lygeia Ricciardi, Ed.M., is an expert and thought leader in consumer engagement and digital health. Her consulting practice, Clear Voice Consulting, helps clients from tech start-ups to large multinationals position themselves strategically and communicate effectively with their customers in the growing consumer digital health marketplace.

Previously Ms. Ricciardi established and directed the Office of Consumer eHealth at the Office of the National Coordinator for Health Information Technology, where she led the Blue Button Initiative and integrated the consumer perspective into Meaningful Use requirements and other federal policies and programs. She has also worked at start-ups, Harvard Business School, the Markle Foundation, and the Federal Communications Commission. Ms. Ricciardi has been voted among the "Top 10 Most Influential Women in Health IT" and featured by C-SPAN, the *Wall Street Journal*, and National Public Radio.

Rebecca Schnall, Ph.D., RN, has focused her work on persons living with or at high risk for HIV/AIDS (PLWHA), a disease that affects nearly 1.2 million Americans. Dr. Schnall's research has informed New York state policy. Through federally funded research, she explored the use of informatics tools used in the implementation of the New York state HIV testing law. Her research team found that while electronic alerts increase testing rates, they do not increase the diagnosis rates of HIV. This work, published in peer-reviewed journals and presented at national and international conferences, continues to influence policy makers and clinicians in the implementation of other mandatory health screening programs.

In addition, Dr. Schnall's research guides public health efforts to improve population health at the national level. She recently completed a Centers for Disease Control and Prevention (CDC)-funded project to inform the design of mobile applications for HIV prevention and treatment. The information from that study is foundational to CDC's prevention efforts of HIV in high-risk men who have sex with men. Findings will also be used to inform the development of a CDC mobile application for PLWHA for the management of their disease. This study is one of the first attempts to identify the functional components and information that should be contained in an app from HIV persons and their care providers. This important work will also contribute to the knowledge base for developing informatics tools and strategies in building mobile applications that can be extended to the development of mobile health technology for managing other chronic illnesses.

Dr. Schnall's work in the field of informatics has also contributed to the development of self-management tools for chronically ill patients. She led a feasibility study to design and test a Web-based symptom self-management tool for PLWHA. Findings from the study demonstrated the feasibility and usefulness of Web-based tailored systems for decreasing symptom frequency and intensity in PLWHA. Finally, she has contributed to the science of informatics by developing and refining innovative informatics methods to understand the usability factors associated with the use of mobile health technology. Her work has demonstrated novel methods for assessing the usability of mobile devices and validated the use of a new usability evaluation framework for mobile health technology. Importantly, these contributions have been widely disseminated and contributed to the development of informatics knowledge.

Ted Vickey is the founder and president of FitWell, Inc., a fitness and wellness consulting company specializing in innovation and emerging technology. He is also currently completing a Ph.D. in Engineering, focusing on interdisciplinary research within exercise science, technology, and social networking, at the National University of Ireland at Galway. He is an emeritus member of the Board of Directors for the American Council on Exercise, the largest nonprofit accredited certification organization in the fitness industry.

Prior to his recent studies, Mr. Vickey was vice president of Comprehensive Health Services, where he led the fitness and wellness division of the largest privately held occupational medicine company in the United States.

From 1994 to 2005, he was the executive director of the White House Athletic Center, the fitness center serving the fitness, health, and wellness needs of the staff at the Executive Office of the President under the Clinton and Bush administrations. He has also consulted with companies and organizations such as the White House, Department of Commerce, Securities and Exchange Commission, Fruit of the Loom, Transportation Security Administration, Sylvania, and Allied Irish Bank.

Mr. Vickey holds a B.S. in Exercise Science from Pennsylvania State University and a master's of Business in International Business and Entrepreneurship from the University of Limerick. He frequently presents on fitness and technology to diverse audiences around the world and is the author of four books and numerous academic papers.

Winston F. Wong, M.D., M.S., serves as Medical Director, Community Benefit, Kaiser Permanente, and is responsible for the organization's partnerships with communities and institutions in advancing population management and evidence-based medicine, with a particular emphasis on safety net providers and the elimination of health disparities. As a Captain of the Commissioned Corp of the U.S. Public Health Service from 1993–2003, Dr. Wong was awarded the Outstanding Service Medal. Dr. Wong currently has served on a number of national advisory committees, including those sponsored by the National Quality Forum, Centers for Medicare & Medicaid Services, and the Institute of Medicine (IOM) addressing issues of access and quality for diverse populations, most recently as a member of the IOM Committee on the Integration of Primary Care and Public Health. In 2013, Dr. Wong was appointed to the IOM's Board on Population Health and Public Health Practice. He is also a Board member of The California Endowment, the Essential Hospitals Institute, and the School Based Health Alliance. Bilingual in Cantonese and Toisan dialects, and a graduate of UC

Berkeley and the UC San Francisco School of Medicine, Dr. Wong continues a small practice in Family Medicine at Asian Health Services, a federally qualified health center based in Oakland, where he previously served as Medical Director. Dr. Wong was featured as a "Face of Public Health" in the May 2010 issue of the *American Journal of Public Health*.